Interm Fasting for Women Over 50

(and not only)

JULIA CHRISTEN

Copyright © 2019 Julia Christen

All rights reserved.

OTHER BOOKS BY JULIA CHRISTEN

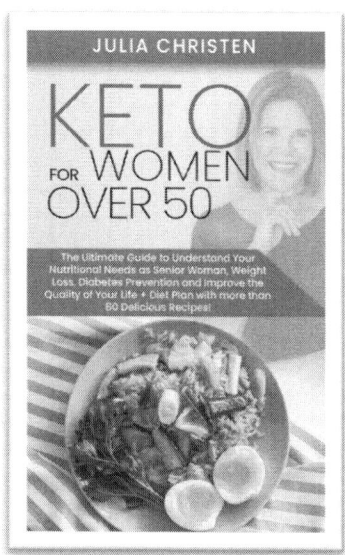

#1 Best Seller

The Ultimate Guide to Understand Your Nutritional Needs as Senior Woman, Weight Loss, Diabetes Prevention and Improve the Quality of Your Life + Diet Plan with more than 80 Delicious Recipes!

Find it on Kindle Store
CLICK HERE

TABLE OF CONTENTS

Introduction 1

Chapter One 3

What is Intermittent Fasting? 3

    The Autophagy Process 7

    The 12/12 Fast 9

    The 16/8 Fast 10

    The 20/4 Fast 11

    5:2 Day Fasting 11

Chapter Two 13

Why Intermittent Fasting is Ideal for Women Over 50 13

    Weight Loss 13

    Metabolic Reset 14

    Increase Human Growth Hormone 14

    Convert Your Body Fat 15

    Improve Muscle Health 15

    Boosted Energy 16

    Reduce Insulin Resistance 17

    Reduce Excess and Chronic Inflammation 17

    Increase Neural Cells 18

    Boost Cellular Health 19

    Lessen Oxidative Stress 20

Improve Mental Well-Being 20
Treat or Prevent Disease 21
Polycystic Ovary Syndrome (PCOS) 21
Non-Alcoholic Fatty Liver Disease 22
Diabetes... 23
Alzheimer's Disease 24
Cancer.. 25

Chapter Three 27

The Pros and Cons of Intermittent Fasting..........................27

The Positives of Intermittent Fasting......................................28

1. Boost Weight Loss 28
2. Balance Important Hormones 29
3. Improve Heart Health... 30
4. Increase Mental Energy and Efficiency............................ 31
5. Reduce the Potential Risk of Developing Cancer............ 32
6. Increase Longevity 33
7. Lifestyle Ease 33

The Potential Downsides of Intermittent Fasting.................34

1. Getting Started Takes an Adjustment 34
2. Potential to Overeat 34
3. Possible Leptin Imbalance 35
4. You May Become Dehydrated.. 35
5. Not Everyone Can Practice Intermittent Fasting 36

Chapter Four 37

Busting the Myths About Intermittent Fasting 37

Fasting Induces Starvation 37

Fasting Causes Lean Muscle Loss 38

Humans Can't Survive Without Water 39

It is Healthier to Eat Small Frequent Meals 39

The Brain Will Be Starved of Glucose 41

Fasting Results in Binge Eating and Weight Gain 41

Fasting Reduces Athletic Performance 42

Fasting Can Damage Health 43

Chapter Five 45

Tricks to Succeed with Intermittent Fasting 45

Research, Research, Research 45

Understand Your Motivation 46

Slow and Steady Wins the Race 46

Drink Plenty of Water 47

Avoid Temptation 48

Enjoy the Caffeine Boost 48

Stay Busy 49

Liberally Season Your Food 50

Prioritize High-Quality and Consistent Sleep 50

Track Your Progress 51

Avoid Fasting When Stressed 52

Chapter Six 55

Enjoying a Balanced Diet with Intermittent Fasting 55

Chapter Seven **63**

Pairing Intermittent Fasting with the Ketogenic Diet for the Ultimate Lifestyle 63

    Foods to Avoid 67

        Grains 67

        Starchy Vegetables and Legumes 68

        Sugary Fruits 69

        Milk and Low-Fat Dairy Products 69

        Cashews, Pistachios, and Chestnuts 70

        Most Natural Sweeteners 70

        Alcohol 71

Chapter Eight **73**

How to Exercise While Fasting 73

Chapter Nine **81**

Recipes 81

Breakfast 83

    Sweet Potato and Chickpea Hash 85

    Oatmeal Pancakes 89

    Keto Burrito Wrap with Bacon and Avocado 91

    Keto Blueberry Pancakes 93

    Keto Sausage and Cheese Vegetable Frittata 95

Keto Cheese and Sausage Scones 97

Lunch 99

Shrimp Greek Salad 101

Sweet Pepper Nachos 103

Spaghetti Squash Garlic Noodles with Chicken 105

Keto California Roll Bowls 109

Keto Chicken Avocado Salad 111

Dinner 113

Big Mac Salad Bowl 115

"Stuffed" Cabbage Casserole 119

Keto Chili 121

Creamy Artichoke Spinach Soup 123

Dessert 125

Keto Chocolate Mousse 127

No-Bake Peanut Butter Pie 129

Berries with Ricotta Cream 131

Conclusion 133

Introduction

Whether you are hoping to lose weight or gain health benefits, many fad diets that claim they can help. Yet, these fads are nothing more than crash diets that cause a person to lose weight overly quickly in an unsustainable manner. The result? A woman may temporarily lose weight, but, before long, they gain even more weight back as the crash diet damaged their metabolism. Many women fifty and over have had their fair share of these diets, whether it is Weight Watchers, the South Beach Diet, Atkins, or worse yet, even more, extreme options such as the lemonade diet. After years of attempting to gain health and lose weight, many women are left worse off than they started.

Fear not; there is a solution. There is a way to lose weight that is not a crash diet. With intermittent fasting, which has been practiced for centuries all across the world, you can boost your health and rev up your metabolism for the ultimate form of maintainable and lasting weight loss.

Intermittent fasting allows your body to go through the eating cycles it is designed for. The human body has gone through these eating cycles naturally during periods of the day and night throughout history. Whether for religious reasons or only as a basic pattern to everyday life, these short terms of fasting allow the body to burn off the calories you have stored and use the break-in eating to heal itself. Intermittent fasting is great for adults of all ages, but especially for women as they age as it can help their metabolism to recover from years of dieting culture, as well as treating common age-related ailments such as high blood pressure, insulin resistance, and more.

By starting your journey with intermittent fasting, you can enjoy all your favorite foods, experience more energy, increased health, and maintainable weight loss. Within the pages of this book, you will find everything you need to get started and then some.

While reading this book, you will often find references to the Ketogenic Diet. That's why I suggest you read my book **"Keto For Women Over 50"** where you will find a detailed explanation of what the Ketogenic diet is, in addition to **more than 80 recipes**! You can find it in the Kindle Store of Amazon.

Chapter One

WHAT IS INTERMITTENT FASTING?

Intermittent fasting, otherwise known as short-term fasting, is different than the long hours of fasting that comes to many peoples' minds when they hear the word "fasting." While long hours of fasting frequently cause intense hunger, weakness, and deprive the body of essential nutrients, the same is not true of intermittent fasting. With this form of fasting, your body still gains all the nutrients and calories it requires, but it also harnesses the body's natural metabolism to its fullest to increase health and weight loss.

It may seem foreign to practice intermittent fasting, but the truth is that humans already practice short-term fasting while sleeping. That is where the word "breakfast" originates, as it is the meal that breaks our overnight fast. The human body is formed in such a way that periods of short-term fasting allow our health and metabolism to reach its peak. Yet, many people in today's modern society snack and graze, never utilizing the benefits that intermittent fasting has to offer.

Fasting has a long history in everyday practice, medicine, and even religion throughout the world. In this chapter, we will examine intermittent fasting and its roots throughout history so that you can fully understand how to harness it and gain all the benefits it has to offer, both to your health and to your waistline.

While previous health theories before the age of science were not always accurate or helpful, science has recently found that many of these practices have a solid basis. The doctors prescribing various practices for healing may not have understood the science behind why something worked, such as in ancient Chinese medicine, but science is slowly examining these practices and coming to know why they are so useful. One shining example of this is intermittent fasting. Many ancient cultures and religions would prescribe fasting for people who were of poor health, and now through scientific studies, researchers have found that intermittent fasting does have healing proprieties. One of the most famous physicians that prescribed fasting during ancient history was Hippocrates from Greece.

Fasting has also been practiced for religious purposes for centuries. Not only have humans used fasting for religion and health, but it was also a necessary aspect of daily life throughout history. Before modern times, many people would be out working in the fields, workshops, or anywhere else they could make a living. Due to this, they were unable to stop and eat quickly. Instead, the time between their meals would lengthen, turning into a valid fasting window. This intermittent fasting, while not intentional, allowed individuals to attain the health and weight benefits that fasting has to offer. Sadly, due to modern amenities, many people no longer practice regular short-term fasting. But, with the new scientific understanding of intermittent fasting's benefits, more people are beginning to go back to this healthy and natural way of life.

As you can see from the religious fasting examples, there are many different types of fasting. Some individuals abstain from all food and drink, others only abstain from food, and sometimes only specific foods are off-limits. Intermittent fasting is a moderate example of fasting in which a person refrains from all food but is free to enjoy any calorie-free drinks. Although, there are a few forms of intermittent fasting that do allow a person to consume a limited number of calories over a more extended period. We will discuss this fasting in-depth later on.

Intermittent fasting is an effective weight loss option as it not only limits your caloric intake, but it also boosts your metabolism, so you burn off more calories and body fat. Most of the time, humans eat so frequently that our bodies are continually attempting to burn off the calories we have recently eaten. But, when you practice intermittent fasting, you give your body that opportunity to burn off body fat instead of a snack, thereby allowing you to lose weight.

Even if you eat a low-calorie snack, you will likely be adding to your body weight. This is because your body can only hold a certain amount of glucose at one time, and once your glucose reserves in your muscles and liver are full, the body must transform the remaining glucose into lipids, which are stored as body fat. Since low-calorie snacks are made with carbohydrates, which is glucose, whenever you graze on these snacks during the day, you impede your weight loss.

On the other hand, if you eat a large calorie-dense and nutritious meal that will keep you satisfied, you can go all day without eating. This will not only lower your daily calorie intake, but it will also allow you to burn off the calories you consumed in your meal plus your body fat, reducing your weight at a manageable and healthy rate.

There are multiple types of intermittent fasting, which allows a person to find the exact version that is right for their lifestyle. Unlike diets that make you change your lifestyle to lose weight, you will find that intermittent fasting can seamlessly fit into most lifestyles. You can customize the approach to best work for you. There is no need to miss out on dining out with family, going out drinking with friends, or enjoying your favorite foods in moderation.

For instance, if you typically enjoy going out to eat with family and friends in the evening, you can begin your fasting after your last meal or drink, and then fast until noon the following day. This will allow you to enjoy your healthy lifestyle while still practicing intermittent fasting. As many people do not feel hungry in the morning, this is a common approach to intermittent fasting. Of course, you can choose any time of day to fast that best works for you, and you can customize your fasting window length.

When you take up intermittent fasting, you shouldn't have to obsess over food or when you eat or don't eat. You shouldn't be staring at the clock hungry and tired, waiting for your next meal. Instead, you can listen to your body, eat when you are hungry, and go without when you are satisfied. Of course, when you first begin intermittent fasting, there will be an adjustment period, but you can make this easier on yourself by slowly altering your usual eating habits. For instance, if you usually eat every four or six hours, you can gradually increase the time between meals by thirty minutes. By increasing your fasting window by only thirty minutes at a time, you won't suffer from hunger pangs or fatigue, but you will allow your body to adjust to a fasting lifestyle slowly.

When you begin intermittent fasting, it is essential to remember that you don't only increase the time between your meals, but you also eat healthier meals that are calorie-dense. By eating a large number of healthy calories within a meal, you will be able to go more extended periods between eating while still staying satisfied and full.

While you can eat a regular healthy diet without any constrictions when practicing intermittent fasting, you can also increase the health and weight loss benefits by combining intermittent fasting with a ketogenic diet. The ketogenic diet is perfectly paired with intermittent fasting, as it prioritizes healthy and calorie-dense meals. Not only that, but as the ketogenic diet produces the fuel type known as "ketones," which are also produced when fasting, you will find that you experience increased energy.

You must understand that your body is not in a fasted state the entire time you are fasting. When you first finish a meal, your body is in a fed state, also known as the absorptive state, where it is working on breaking down the nutrients you have eaten. After a few hours, you enter the post-absorptive state, in which your body is working to use the food you have eaten as fuel. Lastly, after eight to twelve hours of not eating, you enter the fasted state. During the fasted state, you have burned off the calories from the food you have eaten, and your body will turn to use body fat as a fuel source, as well as producing ketones for fuel. While a short twelve-hour fast can give you health benefits, if you do not enter the fasted state until hour twelve of not eating, then you will only experience a small portion of the health and weight loss benefits intermittent fasting has to offer. On the other hand, a longer fasting window, such as a sixteen-hour fast, will give your body a long time to remain in a fasted state, allowing you to reap all the benefits intermittent fasting has to offer.

THE AUTOPHAGY PROCESS

Autophagy, pronounced as "aw-TOFF-uh-gee," is a vital human metabolic function. Sadly, this function can slow down as we age, causing health numerous health problems for women as they approach age fifty. But, what does autophagy mean? It is a combination of two Greek words, and when placed together, these words translate to "eat thyself."

Most laypeople still have very little to no understanding of the autophagy process, as researchers only began to understand the basics of it back in the 1950's. Yet, what these researchers learned is incredibly valuable. They found that there is a particular aspect of the cells within our bodies known as the organelle, specifically the lysosome organelle. Within the lysosome are enzymes whose express purpose is to aid in the digestion of fuel.

Later on, it was discovered that the lysosome organelle contains within them even smaller cells and organelles. But what does it mean? This shocking revelation spurred the researchers onward, and they found that there is a system, later named autophagosomes, that drive old and damaged cells to the lysosomes.

You may be wondering what the purpose of the autophagy system is and why the lysosome must consume other cells. When our cells become old and damaged, they are no longer able to function correctly. Therefore, the lysosome helps not only by consuming and getting rid of these cells but by recycling them to build and create younger and healthier cells that we can effectively use.

We all use the autophagy metabolic process in our daily lives in ways that we aren't even aware of. For instance, when we have been infected with a virus or bacteria after our immune system works on fighting back against the harmful properties, it is the autophagy process that helps to remove the toxic substances from our system.

This incredibly important system cannot be replicated by the use of prescription drugs, although researchers are seeking to find a way to activate it for the treatment of diseases. Yet, while you are not able to induce it with medication, there is another way to boost and increase your natural autophagy system: by practicing intermittent fasting. By triggering such an increase through fasting, women over fifty can begin to take back their health and prevent age-related diseases such as early-onset Alzheimer's diseases, type II diabetes, cancer, and more.

If you want to age well and feel young again, I can't stress enough the importance of the autophagy system and putting it to work for you.

Now that you have an understanding of the basics behind the fasting method, let's look at the main types of intermittent fasting.

THE 12/12 FAST

The perfect fasting method for beginners is the 12/12 fast, which is named such due to the twelve-hour feeding window and twelve-hour fasting window. When getting started, it may sound like going twelve hours without eating is a lot, but you likely already do this, at least some of the time. After all, if you finish eating your last meal of the day at 7 pm and then eat breakfast at 7 am, you have completed a twelve-hour fast!

If you are someone who habitually snacks late at night, try to prioritize eating more substantial nutrient and calorie-dense meals, which will keep you satisfied until your morning meal. Keep in mind that while this is a beautiful fast to get started with, you will want to try more advanced and longer fasting windows in the future. This is because the human body generally only enters the fasted state after twelve hours without eating, so you will only be able to gain a limited number of benefits with a short fast. To attain the full benefits of intermittent fasting, you will want to advance to a longer fast, such as the 16/8 fast, which will allow you to remain in the fasted state for several hours before eating.

THE 16/8 FAST

One of the most popular fasting methods is the 16/8 fast, named so due to the sixteen-hour fasting window and eight-hour eating window. This method is so popular, as it is simple to accomplish once you have adjusted to intermittent fasting with the 12/12 way. Due to its longer fasting window, you can experience all the benefits of intermittent fasting, as the human body enters the fasted state at around twelve hours after eating, meaning you can stay in the metabolic fasted state for approximately four hours before eating again.

You will find that this method is also known as the Leangains Method, and some people will customize it to have a shorter fasting window. Some women prefer to use a fourteen or fifteen-hour fast instead of the sixteen-hour, but it is all based on personal preference and ease.

While everyone can adjust this fast to their schedule, one common way to practice the 16/8 fast is simply by skipping breakfast. This is easy for many people who find that they are not hungry in the morning. But remember, to skip breakfast, you first have to ensure that you eat a large and healthy dinner the night before to help sustain you until lunchtime.

When lunchtime arrived, don't eat a small or unhealthy meal. Instead, you should focus on eating healthy and calorie-dense food that will refuel your energy and prepare you for the next time you fast.

THE 20/4 FAST

While a more extreme version of fasting, women who have adjusted to the 16/8 fasting method and want more of a challenge may desire to try the 20/4 fast. A large fluid intake must accompany the twenty hours of fasting during the fasting window. During your four-hour eating window, try to eat two large and calorie-dense meals, full of healthy nutrients. You will want these meals to contain your entire caloric, protein, and fat needs for the day.

This fast is often best started after lunchtime. By starting after lunch, you can enjoy a large breakfast, lunch, and maybe even a snack before you begin your fast. If you finish lunch at 12 pm, then your fast will go until the following day at 8 am, meaning you can eat your meals that day as usual.

If you find this fast is overly tricky when you first start, don't hesitate to cut it short. Instead of pushing yourself to finish the full twenty-hour fast, you can slowly increase your fasting window naturally until you get to your goal.

5:2 DAY FASTING

This method of fasting is the most intense that we describe here, as two days out of the week, a person fasts for nearly the entire day.

You should not schedule your two fasting days together, but instead, have them separated by eating days. For instance, don't schedule your fast for both Tuesday and Wednesday. Alternatively, you should schedule them for Tuesday and Thursday so that you have a day in-between to eat plenty.

On fasting days, a person should generally consume only calorie-free drinks, such as water. But women are allowed five-hundred calories in food these days. This means you can have one large meal, prioritizing nutrients such as healthy proteins and fats. This method of fasting should be scheduled on days that are easiest for you. Most people choose to not fast on the weekends, as that is their time to enjoy themselves fully. Instead, weekdays, where you are at work or busy with errands, are often the best days to fast, as you will be too busy to think about eating.

While any of these fasting methods will work for women fifty and over, you want to prioritize a method ideal for the aging female body. While every woman is different, in general, the best option will be a fourteen to sixteen-hour fasting window. With this window, you can experience all benefits that a longer fasting window has to offer, but without the struggle of making it through a prolonged fasting window. You can enjoy slightly more frequent meals to keep your energy up, and still lose weight and boost your health.

Chapter Two

WHY INTERMITTENT FASTING IS IDEAL FOR WOMEN OVER 50

There are many benefits to intermittent fasting that make it ideal for women as they age. Not only do women struggle to lose weight as they get older, and their metabolism slows down, but they also are more prone to many age-related and weight-related diseases. In this chapter, we will go point-by-point on some of the best reasons to choose this lifestyle.

Weight Loss

While many people try diet after diet to lose weight, only to be disappointed, you can expect to find much more success with intermittent fasting. After all, while the human body is usually forced to be burning off the food regularly we have eaten, when you are in a fasted state, you can instead work on burning off your body fat. In the past, it was natural to go long periods without eating while working for the day. In today's modern society, we take a break for lunch and often for a snack as well, which only impedes weight loss. But, with fasting, you can eat the same number of calories and still lose weight, all because you are allowing your body to use the fat it has stored up.

Multiple studies conducted on intermittent fasting have found it much more effective than a variety of popular dieting and weight loss options, even when a person doesn't reduce their caloric intake.

Metabolic Reset

Many women, as they age, experience reduced metabolism. This is partly due to the natural aging process, and partly due to damaging the metabolism over the decades. Frequent crash dieting, poor sleep, overworking, poor health, and more can all damage your metabolism, thus preventing you from losing weight. But, by merely practicing intermittent fasting, you can reset and boost your metabolism, not only allowing you to lose weight but also helping you to feel healthier and maintain healthy lean muscle as you age.

Increase Human Growth Hormone

Hormones play an essential role in human health, something of which women are exceptionally aware of as they age. But many women are unaware of how to take advantage of the human growth hormone, also known as HGH. As this name implies, this hormone affects growth, but that is not all! This hormone is vital for bone health and density, cellular growth and regeneration, tissue health, and muscle mass. As women age, they tend to lose muscle mass, bones become thin and brittle, and cells begin to decay, increasing the speed of aging: all things that an increased level of HGH hormone can help improve.

When your body is in a fasted state, it leads to a boost in a natural increase in the HGH hormone. Studies have proven that this hormone can rise to five times its average level during a fast, meaning you can experience great full-body benefits to your health.

While it can be harmful if you experience a rise of this nature in many of your hormones, the same is not true of the human growth hormones. Studies have found that it is perfectly safe, even when it rises to this degree and higher. This is especially true since people naturally experience their HGH levels lowering as they age.

Convert Your Body Fat

Many people are unaware, but there are two types of body fat, white and brown. This fat is not created equal. Just as there is healthy and unhealthy cholesterol, there is also sturdy and unhealthy body fat. The white fat, which is what builds up as people gain excess weight, is damaging to health, contributes to aging, and leads to disease.

On the other hand, brown body fat is vital in protecting the body's inner organs and maintaining health. When you practice intermittent fasting, it not only helps you lose weight, but it can also actively convert your unhealthy white fat to healthy brown fat. As if that weren't good enough, brown fat also helps burn off white fat, meaning that the more brown fat you have, the more you will burn off excess white body fat.

Improve Muscle Health

Many people get excited about the temporary weight reduction they experience when trying the crash diet. That is until they stop losing weight and eventually give up on a diet. But, most of the weight loss people achieve on these diets is not fat loss but water weight and muscle weight. Muscle weighs more than fat, so even a small amount of muscle loss can make a big difference on the scale.

As crash diets promote malnutrition, it naturally leads to muscle loss, which negatively affects your health and strength as you age. After all, your muscles are in much more than your arms. They are surrounding your entire body, and even your heart is a muscle! As you lose muscle, your health and energy will be dramatically affected, and it is essential to regain this as you age if you want to improve your health. Thankfully, studies have found that when compared to dieting, intermittent fasting not only leads to more weight loss than dieting, but it also causes much less muscle loss. This means your muscles will become much healthier, especially if you actively workout while you practice fasting.

Boosted Energy

The mitochondria, which are within our mitochondrial cells, are the powerhouse of the cell. It is the mitochondria that allow us to use a variety of fuel sources from the food we eat as fuel, as well as ketones. While other cells in the body may only be able to utilize one or two fuel types for energy, the mitochondrial is incredibly versatile to be able to use all kinds of fuel. When you fast for longer periods (or are on a low-carb/ketogenic diet), your body begins to produce ketones, which are then used to cross the blood-brain barrier and fuel the brain in the absence of glucose. But that is not all. When you are in this fasted state of ketosis, the body will also increase the number of mitochondrial cells within your body, replacing non-mitochondrial cells with mitochondrial cells, allowing for more of your cells to be fueled by any fuel source.

Since the mitochondrial fuel ninety percent of the human body, by increasing the number of these cells, you can naturally increase your energy. Not only will your physical energy increase, but your mental functioning and energy will, as well. This is great news for many people who lose energy as they age.

Reduce Insulin Resistance

Insulin is perhaps the most well-known hormone, as the number of people diagnosed with diabetes only continues to rise. But insulin does not only affect people with diabetes but for everyone. This hormone, produced by the pancreas, is released after eating to allow the cells to absorb and utilize glucose as an energy source. But, often, our sensitivity to insulin decreases as we age or put on weight. The cells can become resistant to insulin, which leads to them being unable to absorb the glucose we have ingested. Over time, this causes a buildup of glucose in the bloodstream and, ultimately, diabetes if it is left untreated.

However, whether you have insulin resistance or already have been diagnosed with type II diabetes, you don't have to allow your condition to worsen. You can treat your insulin resistance directly at the source, and in the process, improve the absorption of glucose by your cells. Many people can lower the severity of their insulin resistance or diabetes, and some are even able to treat it completely.

Multiple controlled studies have found that intermittent fasting can both treat insulin resistance and lower blood glucose levels. Some studies have found that intermittent fasting can even be as effective, if not more effective, than dieting for lowering blood glucose levels.

Reduce Excess and Chronic Inflammation

Inflammation plays an essential role in human health. Without inflammation, we would be the victim of any germ or bacteria that attempted to leave our body. This is why people with a compromised immune system can get sick and pass away so easily.

But, while it might be important to have a functioning immune system that will increase inflammation when we are sick or injured, sometimes we develop excess or chronic inflammation, which is also detrimental to our health. Sadly, cases of excessive and chronic inflammation are becoming more wide-spread due to environmental pollutants, overwork, poor diet, sleep deficiencies, and more. When this happens, the chronic inflammation no longer protects a person from diseases but instead predisposes them to more infection. For instance, studies have found that increased levels of inflammation can lead to heart disease, cancer, rheumatoid arthritis, and much more.

However, you don't have to accept the occurrence of excessive and chronic inflammation helplessly. Studies on the matter have found that intermittent fasting can drastically reduce chronic inflammation levels. One study found that within as little time as a month, participants' inflammation levels were drastically reduced. Another study specifically found that you can achieve these results simply by completing a daily twelve-hour fast for thirty days.

Increase Neural Cells

It is important to take care of brain health as we age, especially as the levels of Alzheimer's disease, Parkinson's disease, and other neurodegenerative diseases are on the rise. But, one way that intermittent fasting can help guard against and treat all brain-related diseases is by increasing the production and repair of neural cells. This is important, as these diseases all cause these vital brain cells to become damaged or stunted overtime.

The result is that if you begin practicing intermittent fasting regularly now, you can reduce your risk of developing a neurological disease in the future. Or, if you already have one, you may be able to reduce symptoms or halt its progression. This is amazing news, as neurological diseases are incredibly hard to treat, even with modern medicine. Studies have specifically shown intermittent fasting to increase cell growth and repair in the cortex, hippocampus, basal forebrain, and nervous system. Along with the decreased risk of disease and disease progression, you can also expect to experience increased mental energy, better focus, improved memory, and a stabilized mood.

Boost Cellular Health

As we age, our cells themselves also age and decrease in age, which is the aging process that we are all so familiar with. But there is a process known as autophagy that can reduce the aging of the cell, and therefore help slightly reduce aging and significantly increase health. There is no method to stop or reverse aging itself, but you can stop and reverse the aging of the cells. The autophagy process causes old, damaged, and dying cells to be replaced with younger and healthier cells, allowing you to maintain health. The process of autophagy is critical for maintaining homeostasis, and if it is malfunctioning, it leads to increased aging and disease.

Researchers have long studied this process, even going to far as to search for drugs that can induce the process of autophagy to treat people with chronic and terminal illnesses. But you can induce autophagy without drug treatments with intermittent fasting. Studies have found that by activating the autophagy process, intermittent fasting can even help your vital stem cells to regenerate themselves.

Lessen Oxidative Stress

Toxins cause oxidative stress. We can develop these toxins when we breathe in poor quality air, don't sleep well, eat poor quality food, apply damaging substances to our skin, and much more. We even develop this oxidative stress when our cells convert fuel to energy, meaning that even if we live in a clean environment, sleep perfectly, and only eat organic food, we would still develop oxidative stress, thereby causing damage to our cells. As our cells develop this damage from oxidative stress, we slowly lose our health and energy, producing an increased risk of disease.

However, studies have shown that intermittent fasting not only increases the rate our cells develop oxidative stress, but it also increases our body's natural antioxidants to fight against this damage directly.

Improve Mental Well-Being

Poor mental health is becoming more common than ever, with over forty-million Americans suffering from one form of mental illness or another, and many others struggling with short-term depression and anxiety. One of the most common causes of disability in middle-aged Americans (as well as those who are young) is chronic severe depression. Yet, a majority of these people never seek professional help.

While I urge you always to seek professional help for your mental health, you can also practice intermittent fasting. Studies have found that with short-term fasting, people can significantly improve their everyday mood, tranquility, alertness, and even the feeling of euphoria. Not only that but also the symptoms of severe depression can be improved with fasting.

Treat or Prevent Disease

While we cannot guarantee that intermittent fasting will prevent you from developing a disease or treat an infection you already have, many studies have proven that fasting can help. These studies have shown that fasting a person can menage their symptoms, possibly reverse the condition, and significantly reduce your likelihood of ever developing a disease. Now that we have looked at the general ways in which intermittent fasting can improve your health, let's have a look at some of the specific diseases and conditions you can expect short-term fasting to improve.

Polycystic Ovary Syndrome (PCOS)

One common condition that affects women around the world, and the most prevalent of the endocrine disorders, is polycystic ovary syndrome. Though, you may know of this condition as the abbreviated PCOS. This condition causes a myriad of symptoms, such as fatigue, obesity, menstrual irregularity, infertility, insulin resistance, body hair, and more. These symptoms can only worsen as a woman age and go through menopause. Yet, despite how it affects the lives of so many women, doctors have to pinpoint the cause of this disorder. So far, it is only believed that genetics, insulin resistance, and excessive chronic inflammation can all contribute to the development and progression of this disorder.

While much still needs to be learned about both this disorder and its treatment, controlled scientific studies have revealed that intermittent fasting can greatly improve a person's life with PCOS. These studies have shown that when a woman practices regular short-term fasting paired with healthy nutrition, she can experience an improvement in many symptoms.

It is worth mentioning that the ketogenic diet has also been shown to be an especially helpful treatment option for women with PCOS, meaning that when you combine this diet with intermittent fasting, you can expect to improve your symptoms even further. In the studies on the ketogenic diet, it was found that not only did intermittent fasting improve overall symptoms, but previously infertile women were able to conceive.

Non-Alcoholic Fatty Liver Disease

A common condition in people who have developed excessive body fat, especially when located around the abdomen, is non-alcoholic fatty liver disease. The treatment of this disease is frequently weight loss, which, as you are now well aware of intermittent fasting is ideal for. However, the benefits of intermittent fasting for those with this form of liver disease go beyond just weight loss. After all, while it is most common for people with excessive abdomen fat to develop this disease, a person doesn't even have to be overweight to improve it. This disease is caused when fat builds up in the liver, but for some people, fat will build up in this organ even when they are at healthy body weight, making it even harder to treat. Yet, when fatty liver disease is left untreated, it leads to deteriorating health and may also develop into dangerous liver failure, which requires liver transplantation if the person is to survive.

Intermittent fasting can help because it not only helps you to reduce weight and, therefore, the importance of your liver but also because it changes how your body stores its fat. Through studying fatty liver disease, researchers found that individuals who are more prone to storing fat in their liver also have lower levels of a specific protein gene. The good news is that they also found intermittent fasting increases this protein gene, meaning that your liver is less likely to hold onto fat and more likely to shed excess weight. This can help both people who are currently seeking to rid themselves of non-alcoholic fatty liver disease and those who hope to prevent it in the future.

Diabetes

A person who is experiencing severe diabetes and having to undergo insulin treatment may be unable to practice intermittent fasting. Only your doctor will be able to determine whether or not you can safely practice short-term fasting. But, if your condition isn't as severe and your doctor believes it to be safe in your circumstance, then you will be happy to know studies have found intermittent fasting to be incredibly beneficial. Even if you cannot at this time practice intermittent fasting, you may still be able to improve your health enough through the ketogenic diet, at which time you could also take up intermittent fasting under your doctor's discretion.

As you know, intermittent fasting treats excessive weight gain, insulin resistance, and high blood sugar, so it is clear to see why it would help treat diabetes, which is characterized by these three occurrences. Intermittent fasting is so successful that one recent study even found that it was highly effective for type diabetes II patients who were reliant on insulin injections. The participants in this study practiced their fasting closely under their doctor's care multiple times a week. After a short time following their fasting schedule, they were able to completely reverse their insulin resistance, manage blood sugar levels, reduce excess body weight, and even stop their medication.

Alzheimer's Disease

Something that many of us begin to worry about as we age, especially if we have seen relatives go through it in the past, is Alzheimer's disease. This devastating disease not only separates family members in death but also in life. It separates a person from their very understanding and memory of themselves. Sadly, the rate of people with Alzheimer's disease has only continued to skyrocket over the past few decades, with it now being the sixth leading cause of death. The numbers have risen so much that, between the years 2000 and 2015, the rate of people increased by a shocking one-hundred and twenty-three percent, and it is only continuing to rise.

Sadly, science still does not have an answer on how to stop or reverse the disease. However, it has been shown that intermittent fasting can reduce a person's risk of developing it and lessen the severity. A large part of the reason that intermittent fasting is successful is that Alzheimer's disease consists of a mitochondrial cell dysfunction, although it has many other facets as well, such as dysfunctions in the immune system, protein genes, brain cells, and more. When these dysfunctions occur, it causes plaque to buildup in the neurofibrillary of the brain, causing oxidative stress, excessive chronic inflammation, and further mitochondrial dysfunction. It is a vicious cycle where the symptoms continuously cause the disease to worsen, which in turn makes the symptoms also worsen.

The many components of Alzheimer's disease lead to the brain's neurons becoming insulin resistant, and when they are no longer able to absorb the glucose needed, they can also no longer fuel the cells, leading to cellular starvation and death. But as intermittent fasting repairs mitochondrial cells and increases them in number, it can increase the number of cells able to fuel off of non-glucose fuels. It can also treat the insulin resistance itself and cause the production of ketones to fuel the non-mitochondrial neural cells.

Cancer

Lastly, studies have found that intermittent can reduce your likelihood of developing cancer and help make treatment more successful. As you are aware, intermittent fasting can help treat oxidative stress and cellular damage, both of which cause cancer. By reducing this damage, you can thereby reduce your risk of developing cancer in the future.

But that is not all. While human studies still need to be conducted, a study on mice found that when practicing short-term fasting chemotherapy treatment becomes more successful in targeting and treating both breast cancer and skin cancer. Not only did the chemotherapy itself become more effective, but the mice' immune systems also were better able to fight off the cancerous cells and growths, which is essential as chemotherapy is well-known for reducing a person's immune system drastically.

Chapter Three

THE PROS AND CONS OF INTERMITTENT FASTING

There are pros and cons to every lifestyle. For instance, when you are eating a healthy and nutritious diet, you may lose weight and gain health but be unable to eat all your favorite foods in the amount you would like. On the other hand, when you eat junk food all the time you may enjoy yourself, but you will lose health and gain weight. In the same way, there are naturally both pros and cons to intermittent fasting, and by understanding what they are, you can better manage your lifestyle. Like all things, you will find that these pros and cons are most evened out when intermittent fasting is done in moderation. If a person only rarely practices fasting, then they will, in turn, only experience a few of the benefits. On the other hand, if they practice intermittent fasting overly enthusiastically and for longer periods than healthy, then they will experience more of the drawbacks.

Thankfully, with a balanced intermittent fasting schedule, you can find yourself experiencing many of the benefits and few, if any, of the drawbacks. In this chapter, we will be detailing the pros and cons to make it easier for you to make the most of this lifestyle.

While some pros and cons of intermittent fasting are universal, others can be affected by gender and age. In this chapter, we will be exploring what pros and cons you individually may experience as a woman in or over her fifties.

THE POSITIVES OF INTERMITTENT FASTING

1. Boost Weight Loss

Most people discover intermittent fasting either because they want to lose weight or gain health benefits. But, sometimes losing weight can accomplish both of those simultaneously, as a high body fat percentage can increase high blood pressure, cholesterol, and early mortality. Whether you are hoping to gain these health benefits by losing weight or wish to lose weight to feel more comfortable in your skin, you will love the way that intermittent fasting can boost your weight loss.

Many people struggle to find success in typical diets. This is often due to too many crash and fad diets being designed in a way to trigger rapid and quick weight loss, which is unsustainable. The result is either a weight loss plateau or even weight gain over time. But, with intermittent fasting, you can target stubborn weight that won't go anywhere with diets or healthy eating alone.

The human body naturally does better with having specific windows of time for eating, digesting, and burning off fat. But, with our modern society, many people will graze throughout the day, throwing off the natural windows and impeding weight loss and maintenance. The result is that even when a person eats healthfully and exercise, they can still get stuck in weight loss plateaus or gain excess weight.

When we go back to our natural eating and fasting windows, we can begin to experience the real benefits of natural weight loss and maintenance that the human body is designed to accomplish. Not only do fasting periods help to lower your caloric intake, allowing you to lose weight, but it also allows you to still maintain proper eating and nutrition during your eating windows. You can even still enjoy some of your favorite comfort foods in moderation while losing weight!

Controlled scientific studies on intermittent fasting have regularly found that it is more effective than dieting. Researchers have compared the effects of fasting to a multitude of typical diets, and repeatedly intermittent fasting is more effective. This is mostly because not only does intermittent fasting reduce caloric intake naturally and without effort, but also because it increases a person's metabolism. This means that a person is taking in fewer calories while burning more.

2. Balance Important Hormones

One of the most important hormones for our sleep cycles is melatonin. The human body will naturally produce this hormone at night to help us drift off to sleep and stay asleep until morning. But many people still experience sleep disorders. Whether a person has difficulty falling asleep or staying asleep, it will affect their sleep hormones, and their sleep hormones will, in turn, affect their sleep further. This is why a person's sleep disorder will often become more severe over time. As when a person is not sleeping well, their body will no longer produce melatonin properly, and when this happens, the decrease in melatonin will only exacerbate the problem. This disrupts in a person's sleep, and melatonin not only will make them sleepier, but it will also predispose a person to a variety of diseases and weight gain.

Another hormone that will be affected by fasting is cortisol, also known as the stress hormone. When this hormone is increased, not only will a person feel more stressed out and anxious, they will also gain weight more easily, experience increased fatigue, and have trouble falling asleep at night.

Thankfully, studies have found intermittent fasting can help balance a person's cortisol and melioration levels. It does this in a variety of ways. For instance, it can help to reduce cortisol by balancing and regulating blood sugar levels. By balancing cortisol, it sets off a chain reaction that improves the balance of other hormones, including melatonin. One simple change can benefit many hormones and systems within your body.

3. Improve Heart Health

As we age, we all must take even more care of our heart health. After all, heart disease is the number one killer of both men and women. While most often doctors educate men on the symptoms and warning signs of heart attacks, women are often forgotten, leading to increased risk of death. This means women must be extra vigilant, taking care of their heart health and educating themselves on the warning signs of heart attacks.

One crucial way to increase heart health is to watch your cholesterol. There is not a single type of cholesterol, but several. The two main types include LDL, which is known as the "bad" cholesterol, and HDL, known as the "good" cholesterol. While LDL cholesterol will increase your risk of heart attack and heart disease, HDL cholesterol will protect your heart health and remove LDL cholesterol from your body.

Studies on individuals with a high body fat percentage found that when intermittent fasting is practiced, not only is LDL cholesterol lowered, but the number of blood triglycerides is also reduced. It is important to lower these triglycerides, as they are a form of fatty acids that are the building blocks of cholesterol. When we decrease our triglyceride level, it, in effect, makes cholesterol less harmful and reduces our heart health risks.

High blood pressure is a sign of ill heart health, and long-term high blood pressure will increase the damage to your cardiac health and not only increase the risk of heart attack, but also heart disease, stroke, and more. Sadly, many women struggle to lower their high blood pressure, and as a result, are put on medication. Thankfully, studies have found that intermittent fasting can lower blood pressure to a healthy level. This is because when you are fasting, the body will naturally burn its fat and ketones for fuel, and when it is doing this, the liver is unable to produce harmful substances, such as LDL cholesterol, that raise blood pressure.

4. Increase Mental Energy and Efficiency

We all need mental energy to get through the day. When our mind is sluggish, we are unable to think, accomplish anything, and sometimes we may be unable even to stay awake. We have all had troubles at times focusing on work, completing a math problem, remembering what we have read, and so on. This is all due to a lack of mental energy and efficiency. You may think that intermittent fasting would further reduce your mental state, as hunger makes focusing difficult, but the opposite is exact.

Firstly, when done correctly, intermittent fasting reduces hunger, which means that once your body adjusts, you won't have to worry about hunger pangs distracting you. Intermittent fasting can help to improve your mental energy and alertness by increasing your body's natural production of norepinephrine, also known as adrenaline. This natural chemical is an important neurotransmitter within the body, which allows us to increase mental energy, alertness, and efficiency. While further studies on this aspect need to be completed on humans, studies in rats have found that intermittent fasting increases neural cells and connections within the brain. This increase in connections and cells results in a natural increase in mental agility, thought speed, focus, and neural cell communication.

There is an essential hormone within the brain, known as brain-derived neurotrophic factor (BDNF), and studies have proven that intermittent fasting promotes increased levels of this vital hormone. This is important, as when BDNF levels are low, it results in anxiety, depression, and other mental illnesses.

5. Reduce the Potential Risk of Developing Cancer

Of course, nobody can promise that any lifestyle choice will prevent you from developing cancer in the future. However, studies have found that intermittent fasting can potentially reduce your risk. Further studies are ongoing, but current research through animal studies have proven promising. For instance, it was found that rats with tumors survive longer when placed on fasting schedules than the control group.

A human study found that when people practice intermittent fasting while undergoing chemotherapy treatment for cancer, the adverse side effects such as nausea, weakness, and fatigue are reduced. This means that even if a person does develop cancer, intermittent fasting can still help.

Other studies have found that intermittent fasting may reduce the growth of cancer cells and tumors, increasing the patients' likelihood of survival and overcoming cancer.

6. Increase Longevity

Early studies on animals have found that by including intermittent fasting, an animal can experience an increased lifespan. These studies found that even if animals had a higher body fat percentage than the control group, by including intermittent fasting, they were able to increase their lifespan and longevity.

This makes sense, as intermittent fasting has many health benefits, and when all of these benefits are compounded together, it naturally results in a longer lifespan.

7. Lifestyle Ease

We all want improving health and weight, but it is important also to have an easier lifestyle. When it is difficult to gain health and weight, many of us end up failing, as life is already busy and difficult enough without adding added worry and tasks. If a person cook more, eat more frequently, and always worry about a diet, they are unlike to stick to it, as it is merely is unmaintainable.

But intermittent fasting is not a diet, and it results in a much simpler lifestyle. After all, since you have specific fasting windows, it lessens the amount of food you have to cook and how frequently you have to eat, making life easier. The result is that when you are busy, not only do you not have to cook as regularly, but you also don't have to resort to eating junk food, as you can schedule your fasting windows around when you are most busy.

THE POTENTIAL DOWNSIDES OF INTERMITTENT FASTING

1. Getting Started Takes an Adjustment

Any lifestyle change takes an adjustment, and it can take months for something to become a habit. Naturally, intermittent fasting is quite an adjustment for people who are used to grazing on food throughout the day. This means that if you push yourself to go into an advanced version of intermittent fasting when you first begin, you can become overwhelmed. But if you start slowly and allow your body to adjust in its own time, you will find it happens much more naturally and becomes easy to stick to.

You don't have to deprive yourself of food when you are hungry and suffer through hunger pangs. Instead, practice fasting when you are naturally satisfied and eat when you are hungry. If you slowly increase the length of your fasting window, your body will adjust without difficulty, and before long, your body will discover the eating and fasting windows that the human body is naturally inclined to.

2. Potential to Overeat

While intermittent fasting should naturally reduce caloric intake, if a person pushes themselves to fast when they are overly hungry, it might lead to overeating during their eating window. This is because the person feels hungry for so long when fasting when they can finally eat their body believes it must make up for the calories it missed. The result is that the person either hits a weight loss plateau or even experience increased weight.

Thankfully, this is easy to avoid. If you listen to your body by eating when you are hungry and fasting when you are satisfied, you shouldn't overeat. By practicing eating mindfully and slowly, you can also avoid overeating, and you will become more attuned to your body and know when you have eaten enough and can stop.

3. Possible Leptin Imbalance

The hormone leptin is important as it signals to your body that you are full have no longer need to eat. But when a person practices intermittent fasting, it may temporarily disrupt this hormone's production. However, this is usually only a short-term problem, and once a person's body adjusts to their fasting and eating windows, their leptin will balance itself out.

Typically, a leptin imbalance is only a real problem when a person dives head-first into intermittent fasting and attempt to practice advanced level fasting when they are still only a beginner.

4. You May Become Dehydrated

Many people do not drink enough water. In general, doctors recommend that we drink half of our body's weight in pounds in ounces of water. This means that if you weigh two-hundred pounds, you should be drinking one-hundred ounces of water daily.

Not only do many people not drink enough water as it is, but this can make dehydration worse when a person is practicing fasting. This is because fasting boosts the metabolism, and when your cells are in a metabolic accelerated state, they require more water for fuel. If you are not giving them enough water during periods of fasting, you can quickly become dehydrated. Not only that but when fasting, you are likely to lose a lot of water weight, which can result in dehydration and a deficiency in electrolytes. Make sure that you not only drink plenty of water but also consume enough electrolytes to prevent this. Thankfully, dehydration is easy to avoid if you remain proactive.

5. Not Everyone Can Practice Intermittent Fasting

Intermittent fasting is a beautiful and healthy lifestyle for the general population. After all, the human body is designed for practice periods of fasting naturally. However, not every person can practice fasting. Some people, due to chronic illness, may be unable to participate. Ultimately, you must ask your doctor if you are healthy enough to practice short-term fasting.

For instance, people with severe diabetes, metabolic disorders, or those who are pregnant may be unable to practice fasting, even short-term. Whenever you are making a lifestyle change, it is essential first to discuss the matter with your doctor to determine if it is a healthy choice for you individually.

Chapter Four

BUSTING THE MYTHS ABOUT INTERMITTENT FASTING

With the number of fad and crash diets that have come and gone through the ages, there have grown many misconceptions and myths about intermittent fasting. People believe that it is healthier to eat smaller frequent meals, that fasting induces a starvation state, that it will trigger lean muscle loss and more. Thankfully, these myths are simply that: a myth. In this chapter, we will debunk and bust these myths apart with fact and science, so that you can have full confidence in your new lifestyle to gain health and lose weight.

Fasting Induces Starvation

It is commonly believed that fasting induces starvation, which is unhealthy. But this simply is not true. This misconception is understandable, as the fasted state is also referred to as the starved state. However, medically starvation and fasting are very different. While fasting is natural, controlled, and allows a person to consume still all the nutrients and calories their body requires, the same is not true of starvation. Often, fasting is uncontrolled, and it results in a deficiency in nutrients and calories, leaving a person without the vital fuel, vitamins, and minerals their body requires.

People already fast on a nightly basis while asleep, and when you practice intermittent fasting, you do this more purposefully and for slightly longer periods. You still enjoy large, calorie-dense, and healthy meals, along with plenty of fluids throughout the day.

Fasting Causes Lean Muscle Loss

Once again, this fast take root in the false idea that fasting results in deficient nutrient intake. This isn't true! Sure, long-term fasting in which a person is not consuming the nutrients the human body requires, such as in political hunger strikes, might result in lean muscle loss. But the same is not true of healthy short-term fasting. When you practice intermittent fasting, you will be consuming your daily protein requirements during your feeding window, and this protein will stick with you throughout the day for fuel, ensuring you don't lose muscle mass.

Even if you practice a twenty-hour fast, you won't lose muscle mass if you do it properly by consuming plenty of protein and healthy fats during your eating window. Not only will the protein keep your muscles healthy, but the fat will also be transformed into ketones for added fuel, ensuring that your body does not become weakened.

Scientific studies have found that when athletes fast for twelve to twenty hours, there is no risk of muscle loss. Fasting up to forty-eight hours is generally safe (for healthy individuals) as long as a person refuels with the needed nutrients afterward. Although, intermittent fasting is short-term fasting that never goes longer than twenty-four hours. Keep in mind that when you eat a large meal before your fast, that the protein is not all absorbed within a few hours. Instead, protein takes time to be fully absorbed by the body, ensuring that you have protein for fuel all day long. Different sources of protein also absorb at different rates. For instance, the protein within eggs absorbs at a rate of 2.9 grams per hour, whereas a soy protein shake absorbs at a rate of 3.9 grams an hour. If you eat a large meal such as a calorie-rich salad, including chicken, boiled eggs, cheese, bacon, and nuts as protein sources, you will find that you have more than sufficient protein to fuel you throughout your fast.

Humans Can't Survive Without Water

It is a common misconception that you are unable to drink during periods of intermittent fasting. This isn't true! Sure, some religions abstain from all liquids during fasting, such as Muslims during Ramadan. However, this is not a facet of intermittent fasting. Quite the contrary, individuals are encouraged to drink plenty of water to stay hydrated during their fasting window.

Along with water, you can also enjoy calorie-free drinks such as flavored waters, sugar-free sports drinks, tea, and coffee. Artificial sweeteners and sugar alcohols shouldn't be included during your fasting window, though, so no Diet Coke! Why shouldn't these be enjoyed? Because while they may be zero-calorie, your body still has to digest the sweeteners, which will interfere with your fasting. However, you can enjoy stevia leaf extract, which is an herb. This herb is sweet and can be added to drinks, such as coffee and tea.

It is Healthier to Eat Small Frequent Meals

The myth that it's healthier to eat small frequent meals, rather than a few large meals, has no basis in science. This myth began due to unsubstantiated diets that were popular in the '80s and '90s. When you eat smaller frequent meals, your body is always in a fed state where it is forced to digest and absorb the food you have eaten. Your digestive system never gets a chance to rest, and you are rarely able to burn off your body fat. On the other hand, when you go longer periods between your meal, not only does your digestive system get a break from the constant effort of digesting food, you also get an opportunity to burn off your body fat instead of unneeded food.

Once you adjust to intermittent fasting, you shouldn't even feel the need to snack, as your body will learn that you don't have to be putting more calories always. Instead, you will learn to stay satisfied and energized by the nutrients in large meals. Many people believe that eating small, frequent meals boosts your metabolism while large, infrequent meals slow it, but again, this is not true and has no basis in science. This belief mostly began because people misunderstood how the digestive system works. As the body must expend energy to digest a meal, these people believed that by eating frequently, they could harness this use of energy to promote the burning of calories and body fat. Yet, what these people did not understand is that the energy expended during digestion is not affected by how frequently you eat, but rather how many calories you eat. This means that if you eat 12,000 calories in a day, you will expend the same amount of energy to digest them; whether you eat them in small frequent meals or large, infrequent meals, it doesn't change.

Since the frequency of your meals will not affect the number of calories you burn in a day, instead, it is important to limit calorie intake. Intermittent fasting allows you to restrict your calorie intake naturally while you remain satisfied and consume enough nutrients, allowing you to lose weight. You can further compound this benefit by exercising and incorporating the ketogenic diet.

The Brain Will Be Starved of Glucose

The brain requires glucose for fuel, as fatty acids are unable to pass through the blood-brain barrier to fuel your neural cells. However, this does not mean that your brain will be starved while fasting. You don't have to keep ingesting carbohydrates regularly. In fact, out of the three nutrients of protein, carbs, and fat, the only type that humans can live without is carbohydrates. So, how does the brain need glucose, but we also don't need carbs? Simply, the human body is designed in a way that it can survive without a constant carbohydrate/glucose intake. Since glucose is such an important fuel source, the body has its ways to produce this fuel. When a person has burned off all the glucose within their body, then the process of gluconeogenesis will convert amino acids (protein) into the glucose our cells require. Therefore, as long as you eat enough protein, you will always have enough glucose for your brain cells!

Not only will gluconeogenesis ensure you always have enough glucose, but you require less glucose when in a fasted state than when in a fed state. This is because the body will produce ketones when in a fasted state, which can pass through the blood-brain barrier and be used as fuel for the brain. Not only can ketones be used as fuel for the brain, but also for other cells in the body. This is good news, as ketones are a healthier fuel source that reduces the production of free radicals in the body and increase energy levels.

Fasting Results in Binge Eating and Weight Gain

While it is true that a person can binge eat, and therefore gain weight, while practicing intermittent fasting, this is true of any lifestyle. Intermittent fasting does not cause or promote binge eating, and it is entirely dependent on a person's individual choices.

Actually, as many people adjust to intermittent fasting, their overall hunger reduces, as the body realizes, it doesn't need a constant supply of excessive calories. As a person's desire reduces, so too will the amount of food they consume. When you first begin practicing intermittent fasting, you can reduce the risk of binge eating after a fast by slowly and mindfully eating. Instead of sitting in front of the TV or looking at your phone while you eat, slowly enjoy your meal, appreciating each and every bite. Be sure to drink plenty of water, as well!

You can also reduce the likelihood of binge eating by starting your fasting journey slowly. Don't jump right into doing sixteen-hour or twenty-hour fasts. Instead, start with a twelve-hour fast and gradually increase the length of the fast until you naturally reach your quick length goal.

Fasting Reduces Athletic Performance

Athletes commonly worry about lifestyle changes affecting their athletic performance, and for a good reason. But you will be happy to know that when intermittent fasting is done correctly, it won't interfere with your athletic performance. This is especially good for women as they age, as it is important to remain active in promoting healthy aging.

When you first begin practicing fasting, you may be slightly weaker if you push yourself to start too quickly. But, if you start slowly, listening to your body's natural needs, you should find that your energy levels remain intact. But, even if you do feel slightly weaker, this is temporary and will go away once your body adjusts to the change. Once your body adjusts, you won't lose energy as even when in a fasted state, your body will have stores of amino acids, fatty acids, and ketones to burn for fuel. Not only will your body burn off ingested calories, but also body fat, allowing you to lose weight more effectively than when not fasting.

If you do start to feel a reduction in energy, it is more likely due to dehydration or an electrolyte imbalance. Be sure to ingest your daily recommendation of water electrolytes, no matter what. If you suspect you might have an electrolyte imbalance, your doctor can run a simple blood panel to know for sure.

Fasting Can Damage Health

When all your life you have heard fake "science" promoted by crash diets, it's easy to believe that intermittent fasting might harm your health. But the truth is that independent and controlled scientific studies have time and again found short-term fasting not only to be safe but that it also promotes overall health. You can gain a healthier body weight, lower cholesterol, and triglycerides, manage blood sugar, increase energy, and more.

When done as instructed in this book, intermittent fasting does not cause harm to healthy individuals. Although it is important to note that those with certain chronic illnesses and diseases may be unable to handle intermittent fasting, therefore, discuss this lifestyle change with your doctor, and they will be able to evaluate whether or not your health can handle it.

Chapter Five

TRICKS TO SUCCEED WITH INTERMITTENT FASTING

Intermittent fasting is much easier than people first believe, as you pair your fasting periods with feasting periods full of nutritious and satisfying food. Therefore, you stay full during your fasting period, much unlike the meal skipping that most people experience. As long as you start slowly and allow your body to adjust naturally, it should be a simple process. Although, if you do struggle, you should find that after the first five days, things become easier, as after this period, your body will begin to adjust, and fasting will become routine. In this chapter, we will go over some tips and tricks that can make your intermittent fasting journey easier, helping you to gain success, lose weight, and achieve better health.

RESEARCH, RESEARCH, RESEARCH

It's easy to want to jump right into intermittent fasting once you learn of the benefits it has to offer and humanity's history of naturally including fasting in daily life. But if you jump head-first into a new lifestyle without fully understanding it, you are likely to make mistakes that you will later regret. Instead of starting your fasting journey while only halfway through this book, first read each chapter to gain the knowledge and understanding you need to attain success. Research will be your friend, as when you gain experience, you can avoid mistakes and make the journey easier.

UNDERSTAND YOUR MOTIVATION

Making a lifestyle change when only half understanding your motivation is a setting yourself up to quit halfway through. Any lifestyle change takes effort, and if we only have vague ideas of "I want to be healthier" or "I want to weigh less," we can quickly become defeated at the first sign of hurdles. Instead, sit down and write out a list of attainable goals you hope to succeed with. For instance, what aspects of your health do you want to improve? Do you want to lower your cholesterol? Improve your blood pressure? Manage your blood sugar? Reduce daily fatigue? Reduce insomnia to get two more hours of sleep a night? If you want to lose weight, set yourself both short-term and long-term goals. For instance, in the short-term, you can try to lose ten pounds, but maybe long-term, you want to lose fifty.

By having these goals, you will be motivated to overcome the hurdles that come your way, gaining success, and enjoying a better lifestyle.

SLOW AND STEADY WINS THE RACE

When you are excited about succeeding, losing weight, and gaining health, then it is easy to want to rush into intermittent fasting. After you are armed with all the knowledge you need to succeed, you might want to start right off with a 16/8 or even a 20/4 fast. But this is only setting yourself up for failure, just like the hare in the fable "The Tortoise and the Hare." Instead of seeking the fastest way to your goal, find the most successful approach. What does this mean? Don't jump into the more difficult fasting periods. Rather, start with a 12/12 fast or skipping a meal when you aren't hungry. Just be sure that when you do eat that you eat healthy and nutritious food! You can also start by cutting out snacks and training both your mind and body to not eat between mealtimes. After you adjust to these smaller changes, you can slightly increase your fasting window every few days until you reach your desired fasting length.

DRINK PLENTY OF WATER

The importance of staying hydrated cannot be overstated. The truth is that most Americans do not drink their recommended daily intake, which can lead to headaches, migraines, fatigue, stress, false hunger pangs, and more. In fact, by the time you are feeling thirsty, you already are slightly dehydrated. Don't forget to drink your daily intake of water, which is half of your body's weight in pounds in ounces. This means that if you weigh one-hundred and fifty pounds, you should be drinking seventy-five fluid ounces of water, at least, daily.

When you are dehydrated, you can experience false hunger pangs, making you believe that you need to eat when you don't. If you find yourself feeling hungry during your fasting window, before ending your fast early and eating a snack, instead try drinking a glass of water. If you have trouble remembering to drink water, then keep a reusable water bottle at hand at all times and try using a water tracking smartphone app.

AVOID TEMPTATION

While we may not always avoid being around our favorite tempting foods when possible, don't put yourself in a situation to give in to your cravings. For instance, if you know you have a habit of giving in and eating specific junk foods, try not to keep them at home.

But, avoiding temptation is not always about avoiding your favorite foods, but rather timing when you eat them. For instance, if you have a plan to go out to coffee or for drinks with friends, then don't plan your fast during this time. Instead, work your fast around your schedule so that you can enjoy getting food and drinks with friends without impeding your fasting schedule or weight loss. You can still fully enjoy yourself and experience the benefits of intermittent fasting.

You might also consider tailoring where you go out with friends based on the menu. If you are trying to lower your blood sugar, then instead of going out for ice cream, it would be better for your health to find a healthier alternative until your fasting schedule improves your health. Instead of ice cream, you might choose to go out for coffee or get a slightly healthier dessert option, even.

ENJOY THE CAFFEINE BOOST

If you have high blood pressure, you should watch the caffeine, but if you have normal or low blood pressure, you can generally feel free to enjoy a caffeine boost you help you through your fast. Of course, like all medical decisions, you should ask your doctor about your personalized caffeine intake recommendation.

You will find that caffeine can be especially helpful when you are first adjusting to a fasting lifestyle, as it can reduce appetite, helping you to feel more satisfied between meals. Not only that, but it also will provide you with a nice energy boost.

Just remember not to add anything with calories to your coffee during a fasting window, meaning no sugar, cream, or milk. Save these ingredients for your eating windows, instead. If you dislike black coffee or tea, you can add sugar-free natural stevia sweetener during a fasting window. You can also use sugar-free gum to help reduce cravings during the initial adjustment period.

STAY BUSY

It's easy to think that you don't want to stress while busy, and while you may want to avoid changing lifestyles during stressful periods, it is best to take up intermittent fasting when you are working. After all, many people will snack out of boredom, or at the very least, are more likely to notice hunger pangs when they have nothing but time on their hands. On the other hand, if you stay busy with work, chores, or hobbies, you will be able to get through the fasting period seemingly more quickly, with fewer noticeable hunger pangs or temptations to snack.

Remember, a watched pot never boils, and time seems to move most slowly when you are watching the clock. So, if you fast when you are too busy to notice the hours pass by, you will find that before you know it, your fasting window ends, and you can enjoy your next meal. This doesn't mean you need to take up intermittent fasting when your job is keeping you busy, but at the very least, try to find tasks you can delve into at home to pass the time.

LIBERALLY SEASON YOUR FOOD

Surprisingly to many people, by piling on the seasonings during meals in the way of spices, herbs, and vinegar, you can wake up your taste buds, thereby feeling satisfied and full for longer periods. These ingredients also contain very few calories, meaning you can add them liberally to your dishes without adverse effects on your weight.

In Western countries, many people under season their dishes, as you can tell when you compare typical American or British dishes to those from Asia, the Middle East, and other countries throughout the world. Instead of merely cooking fish or chicken with a little salt and pepper, try using a recipe that uses a handful of different spices, herbs, and vinegar so that you can enjoy a genuinely flavorful dish. Not only will these dishes help keep you satisfied, but you will also find that they taste better and are more enjoyable.

PRIORITIZE HIGH-QUALITY AND CONSISTENT SLEEP

Sleep is a vital part of health and well-being, and that includes our health while practicing intermittent fasting. Not only that but by scheduling your fasting schedule to overlap with your sleeping schedule, you can accomplish a longer fasting window without hunger. Without trying, we all already fast overnight between dinner and breakfast, so with a little knowledge of intermittent fasting, you can make better use of this time.

If you are going to be having a particularly long overnight fast, it can help to go to sleep early so that you do not become tempted to get a midnight snack. Although, keep in mind that some people find that an overly large dinner can interrupt their quality of sleep, so find what best works for both your sleep and your fasting schedule. When leading a busy life, or distracted by a good book or TV show, it is easy to neglect sleep. But you mustn't do this, as when you do not sleep properly, it will alter your hormonal balance. As you become sleep deprived, the hormone cortisol will increase, which not only increases stress and impedes sleep but also increases hunger and weight gain. Leptin and ghrelin will also become unbalanced, further increasing hunger and overeating, thereby blocking your progress.

Only by prioritizing consistent and high-quality sleep, you can significantly increase your success in fasting, but also improve your overall health and weight.

TRACK YOUR PROGRESS

While you shouldn't obsess or hyper-focus on your fasting schedule and results, as this can make people overly stressed and self-conscious, it is important to at least track the basics of your progress. This is because it can sometimes feel like we are not making any progress as the scale is not moving, and then you realize you are actually down two jean sizes. The range is not always accurate; what is more important is how fat is positioned on your body.

Therefore, don't only weigh yourself, but also measure your stomach, hips, waist, bust, chest, upper arms, forearms, thighs, and calves. You don't have to worry about tracking these measurements or your weight daily, but at least monitor them once every week or every two weeks. And remember, when you do check your weight and measurements, write it down to keep a record!

By tracking your progress, not only will you be able to recognize your achievement better as you are making it, but you will also come to understand your body and its patterns better.

You can track your progress in a small notebook, journal, yearly planner, or there are even several of helpful smartphone apps created for this purpose.

AVOID FASTING WHEN STRESSED

We all have times in our life when everything seems to be going wrong. Perhaps a loved one is in the hospital, something happened to a beloved family pet, or you are going through a breakup. Generally, these are not good times to begin a new lifestyle. Sure, sometimes you may not be able to avoid it if you need to improve your heart health or blood sugar, but if you can help it, try to begin intermittent fasting when life does feel like a burden. If you do choose to practice fasting during these times, offer yourself kindness and compassion. You can practice shorter fasting windows rather than going for more advanced fasting windows. Allow yourself to have a comforting treat from time to time. If you mess up, forgive yourself.

When making a lifestyle change, you must practice self-kindness if you hope to succeed.

Chapter Six

ENJOYING A BALANCED DIET WITH INTERMITTENT FASTING

Eating a balanced diet is much more than simply eating a salad. This is especially true when you are practicing intermittent fasting, as you need to ensure that you are consuming the proper amount of both macronutrients and micronutrients. But what are these nutrients? Simply macronutrients are the fuel your body consumes in a larger number, including protein, fat, and carbohydrates. On the other hand, micronutrients are equally essential but consumed in a smaller quantity. Micronutrients typically include vitamins, minerals, and phytonutrients found within plants. While a salad may offer you some vegetables, if you don't pair it with plenty of protein and fat, you will be depriving your body of necessary fuel. Not only that, but many people make simple salads with only lettuce, which is low on the nutrition scale. You are much better off consuming a variety of fruits and vegetables to absorb all the micronutrients your body requires. In this chapter, we will examine how you can enjoy a healthy and balanced diet with intermittent fasting.

Salads are a go-to choice for many dieters because they are low in calories and contain vegetables. However, when you are practicing intermittent fasting, you must ensure you consume all the calories and nutrients your body requires during your feeding window, and a simple romaine salad with ranch dressing will not do that. Yet, all salads are not created equal. For instance, you may choose to eat a roasted chicken thigh with a kale salad topped with roasted beets, fresh avocado, toasted almonds, goat cheese, apple, and a rich olive oil vinaigrette. If you make a meal such as this, you will be consuming plenty of protein, healthy fats, and a variety of essential fruits and vegetables. Not only will this meal provide you with the macronutrients and micronutrients your body requires, but it will also leave you full and satisfied for hours to come.

Remember: Don't focus on low-calorie food, but rather nutrient-dense and satisfying meals. This applies whether you are on a standard healthy diet, or if you are pairing the ketogenic diet with intermittent fasting.

Not only do fruits and vegetables offer you a variety of micronutrients that the body requires, but meat can be quite nutritious, as well! While it is important to enjoy red meat in moderation, it has such a high degree of vitamins and minerals that the occasional serving can be incredibly beneficial. Beef is a prime example of nutritious red meat. Beef consists of twenty-six percent protein, which means that for every one-hundred grams of meat you eat, you can get twenty-six grams of vital protein and amino acids to fuel your body throughout your fast. On average, a serving of beef is considered three ounces of meat, which contains twenty-two grams of protein in total. While beef may contain saturated fats, which should be consumed in moderation, it also has other important and healthy fats such as oleic acid, which is commonly found in avocados and olives, palmitic acid, and stearic acid.

The micronutrients in beef, meaning vitamins and minerals, are essential for the human body. However, many of these nutrients are not well absorbed from plant-based sources. We may absorb a small number of the vitamins and minerals we eat from a salad or roasted vegetables, but the human body absorbs these mispronunciations much more effectively from meat. Let's have a look at some of the micronutrients found in large number within beef:

- **Vitamin B12**
  B vitamins are essential for human health, including vitamin B12. This vitamin helps manage our nervous system, neural health, and is used in the formation of blood. But, unlike some of the other B vitamins, B12 can only be found in animal-derived ingredients, such as meat.

- **Vitamin B6**
  Humans need vitamin B6 in larger quantities than some of the other B vitamins, as it plays an important role in the formation of blood. Without enough B6, we become anemic.

- **Iron**
  There are two different types of iron, and it is very important to consume these to prevent anemia. The first type is non-heme iron, which is found in plant-based ingredients. When you consume non-heme iron in plants such as spinach, your system is unable to absorb and make use of a large portion of the iron, making most of it go to waste. On the other hand, meat, such as beef, contains heme iron, which is easily absorbed and utilized by the body. Some people, no matter how much plant-based non-heme iron they consume, will remain anemic and require heme iron from meat to prevent this condition.

- **Selenium**
  Humans only need a small amount of selenium in their diets, but it is hard to come by. Without enough selenium, our metabolism, thyroid function, and immune system all suffer. Thankfully, with beef, you can ensure you are consuming enough selenium without absorbing too much, as can happen with some other sources of selenium.

- **Zinc**
  An essential micronutrient for the immune system, zinc keeps us healthy by fighting off germs such as those that cause the flu and everyday cold. Often, when a person experiences a large number of viral infections, it is due to insufficient consumption of zinc. While there may be supplements on the market of zinc to help you when you come down with a cold, the human body better absorbs this mineral when you consume it in your everyday diet, such as in beef. Not only that, but you will also find it more useful to consume adequate levels of zinc regularly than only when you are sick. This way, it can help prevent you from coming down with illnesses in the first place.

- **Creatine**
  A vital antioxidant, creatine helps us to maintain muscle health, maintain bone density, improve neural functioning, and increase the functioning of our inner organs. Creatine can also increase energy levels, meaning it can help boost your energy when you are adjusting to the intermittent fasting lifestyle.

- **Taurine**
  This nutrient is commonly found within both meat and fish, and it is important for heart and blood health, which

is especially helpful for women as they age. Studies have found that taurine can be especially helpful in the treatment of congestive heart failure, cystic fibrosis, and other heart and blood-related illnesses.

- **Niacin**
  Also known as vitamin B3, niacin is used throughout the human body for basic functioning. Put simply, without niacin, humans could not survive. But this is good news, as by consuming foods rich in niacin such as beef, chicken, salmon, and tuna fish, you can improve many aspects of your health. Niacin is primarily known to help manage heart and brain health, which are two of the most important aspects to focus on as we age.

- **Glutathione**
  One of the most powerful antioxidants known is glutathione. While this antioxidant can often be found in the peel on grapes and wine, one of the most under-rated sources of glutathione is meat. While you can benefit from this antioxidant in any source of beef, you will find that grass-fed beef contains the highest levels of this nutrient and others.

As you can see, there are many reasons to consume meat, as it has many nutrients. Beef is just one prime example. Other meats, such as fish, also offer several micronutrients while having less saturated fats that can raise cholesterol. When consuming fish, the best sources are smaller fish high in fat. The fat in fish is high in omega-3 fatty acids, which most people in Western countries do not consume enough of. This is detrimental, as when we consume low levels of omega-3 and high levels of omega-6 fats, it causes inflammation and increases the risk of disease. But, by lowering your omega-6 intake and increasing your omega-3 consumption, you can greatly improve your health. Fatty fish such as salmon and sardines are two of your best options.

Try to avoid larger fish options, such as tuna, as the larger a fish, the higher mercury contamination it contains. This is because larger fish eat smaller fish, thereby increasing their mercury contents, and when you eat these fish, the mercury contamination crosses over to you. Sardines are one of the best options, as they are rich in omega-3 fatty acids, and since they are small, they contain very little mercury. Sardines are also inexpensive and sold in tin cans, making them stay shelf-stable for long periods. If you purchase bone-in sardines, you can also benefit from an increase in calcium for bone health.

As you can see, both meat and fish have many health benefits. Healthy eating goes beyond eating just fruits and vegetables, but it is about everything you eat. To eat a balanced diet is important to choose a balance of healthy proteins, fats, and carbohydrates. Of course, you do not need to consume many carbohydrates, as this is the one fuel source the body does not require through consumption. The ketogenic diet, which is extremely low carb, can further increase the health benefits you receive through intermittent fasting and boost weight loss. The ketogenic diet can also make intermittent fasting easier, and it prioritizes protein and fat consumption and increases the production of ketones.

When possible, try to choose grass-fed and organic ingredient options, as these not only don't contain harmful substances, they also provide more nutrition. For instance, studies have found that grass-fed butter contains an average of five times the nutrients of grain-fed butter. This increase of nutrients carries over to everything you eat, whether animal-based or plant-based.

It is okay if you can't afford to buy all your ingredients organic and grass-fed, but when you are able, it is best to budget some of your ingredients to at least be higher quality. The best foods to prioritize as organic and grass-fed include meat and vegetables and fruits on the dirty dozen list. The dirty dozen list is fruits and vegetables that contain the highest level of contamination from harmful substances, and therefore are safest to buy organic. This list includes:

- Strawberries
- Spinach
- Nectarines
- Apples
- Peaches
- Pears
- Cherries
- Grapes
- Celery
- Tomatoes
- Sweet bell peppers
- Potatoes

While the ketogenic diet pairs well with intermittent fasting, not everyone chooses to combine the two lifestyles, and that is okay. If you decide to not go on the ketogenic diet, then be sure to prioritize the quality of the carbohydrates you are consuming, as well. You don't want to eat tons of fruit, which is high in glucose and fructose. Fruit is good in moderation, but remember that sugar is sugar, whether it is coming from fruit or cane sugar.

It is best also to choose whole grains rather than processed grains, as the fiber content is higher. This is important, as fiber improves digestive health, allows your body to absorb nutrients better, removes harmful cholesterol from the body, and helps you to remain full and satisfied for longer periods. On the other hand, processed grains that have had most of their fiber removed will spike your blood sugar and in turn, cause a blood sugar crash, making you feel hungry and tired.

When choosing sources of fat, remember that not all fat is created equal. You should prioritize monounsaturated fats such as those in olives, avocados, and nuts. These are the healthiest sources of fats. The second-best source of fat is polyunsaturated fats, which you can find in seeds, walnuts, fish, safflower oil, and soy-based products. The saturated fats found in meats and coconut oil can raise cholesterol, and therefore should be eaten in moderation. Yes, you can enjoy beef and other meats as they have nutritional benefits, but remember always to prioritize the healthier fats over saturated fats. For instance, instead of eating full-fat meat, you may purchase a lower-fat cut off percentage of ground beef and alternatively add fat to your meal with olive oil, avocado oil, or toasted nuts. This will ensure you can both get the nutrients in meat while also prioritizing the best sources of heart-healthy fat.

Chapter Seven

PAIRING INTERMITTENT FASTING WITH THE KETOGENIC DIET FOR THE ULTIMATE LIFESTYLE

Intermittent fasting can be taken to the next level when you pair it with the ketogenic diet. But what is the ketogenic diet? It is a method of eating developed by doctors and researchers a century ago to treat neurological health conditions, such as epilepsy. Over the decades, the method has been improved upon and undergone countless studies. These studies have found that not only does the ketogenic diet improve neurological health, but it also helps heart health, increases weight loss, and more.

The ketogenic diet is a method in which a person consumes very few carbohydrates (on average, twenty-five or fewer net grams a day) and instead prioritizes the consumption of healthy protein and fats. Due to limiting carbs while increasing fats, the ketogenic diet triggers the body to produce ketones as a fourth fuel source. Ketones are also produced when a person practices fasting. This means that when you practice the ketogenic diet, you will already be producing ketones on a constant basis, allowing your body to stay energized and full the entire time you are fasting, as your body is already used to utilizing this energy source. In this chapter, we will explore how you can benefit from pairing the ketogenic diet with intermittent fasting if you so choose.

When the human body is in a fasted state, the mitochondrial cells, with the mitochondria being the powerhouse of the cell, begin to produce ketones. These are a fuel source that, unlike fat, can cross the blood-brain barrier to fuel the neurons in the absence of glucose. But, not only are these ketones produced during a fasted state, but also on the ketogenic diet as the mitochondrial cells will begin producing them upon realizing that your diet is low in carbohydrate and, therefore, glucose.

While the ketogenic diet and fasting have some benefits unique unto themselves, they also share some of the same benefits. Because of this, when you combine the ketogenic diet and intermittent fasting, you can compound upon the benefits for even greater success. For instance, you can expect to experience healthier cholesterol and blood sugar levels sooner than you would by using either the ketogenic diet or intermittent fasting along. Of course, you can also expect to lose weight more quickly, as well.

Many people pair the ketogenic diet and intermittent fasting together, as the high fat and protein contents on the ketogenic diet are ideal to stay full, satisfied, and energized during long periods of fasting. Plus, with the absence of carbohydrates, you won't have to struggle with blood sugar highs and lows during your fasting window. When practiced alone, both the ketogenic diet and intermittent fasting are powerful but paired together; they are an amazing and unstoppable powerhouse.

While you may be able to enjoy foods such as whole-grains, beans, and fruits while you are solely practicing intermittent fasting, this will change if you combine fasting with the ketogenic diet. As you will be eating so few carbohydrates in a day, you will be avoiding grains, beans and legumes, high-starch vegetables, and most fruits. There are a few fruits that can be enjoyed in moderation, such as berries, but most fruits are overly high in sugar. Along with avoiding any carb-heavy ingredients, you will also want to avoid unhealthy fats and instead prioritize the consumption of healthy fats. Remember, since the ketogenic is high in fat, if you eat a large number of unhealthy fats, you can expect it to be detrimental to your health, just as it negatively affects your health when you eat sugary and fried foods. So, instead of eating anything that has a high-fat content, instead choose healthy monounsaturated and polyunsaturated fats in general, with saturated fats from dairy, meat, and coconut in moderation.

When on the ketogenic diet, it is important to keep in mind that there are two types of carbohydrates that you will be calculating: total carbs and net carbs. As you read a nutritional label of a given ingredient, you will always see the total carb count, and sometimes it might even list the net carb count. While you can typically only eat twenty-five carbs on the ketogenic diet, this is a net carb limitation, not a total carb one. But the good news is that even if a nutrition label doesn't list the net carbs, you can easily calculate it yourself!

So, what is the difference between total and net carbs? Net carbs have removed the calculation for any carbohydrates that are not processed by the body and, therefore, won't affect your blood sugar. Most of the time, this calculation removes fiber, but it can also remove sugar alcohols.

As the body does not digest fiber, it will not affect your blood sugar, insulin, or calorie consumption. But fiber is still a form of carbohydrate, which is why it is included in the total carb calculation. Sugar alcohols are a natural sweetener, that much like fiber, are not processed by the body. During the process of digestion, the body is unable to digest sugar alcohols and, therefore, will excrete them, ensuring they don't alter your blood sugar, either. This is why many natural sweeteners, such as Truvia and Swerve, are calorie-free.

If you were to calculate the net carbs in a single serving of strawberries, you would look at the total carb count, which is eleven, and then the dietary fiber count, which is three. When you remove the fiber count from the total carb count, you are left with the net carb count: eight.

You will find that there are many keto-friendly products on the market that use sugar alcohols such as erythritol and xylitol as sweeteners. Along with these two sugar alcohols, the products might also contain stevia leaf extract and monk fruit extract, both of which are also keto-safe. Often, these products will contain the calculated net carb count making it easy on the consumer, as they are marketed to those on a low-carb diet.

The amount of protein a person needs on the ketogenic diet varies based on their body type, activity level, and gender. But, in general, the ketogenic diet focuses on moderate protein consumption, with it making up an average of twenty to twenty-five percent of your diet. Some people may boost their protein intake up even further, to thirty percent, if they are interested in weightlifting and muscle building. It is important to consume adequate protein; otherwise, you will experience lean muscle loss, a weakened immune system, and be at a higher risk of developing common diseases. Thankfully, it is easy to consume enough protein in your daily diet between enjoying meat, fish and seafood, dairy, seeds, nuts, tofu, and eggs.

To know exactly how much you should be eating of the macronutrients (carbs, protein, and fat), you should be eating on the ketogenic diet. You should calculate your macros. Thankfully, this is made easy with online keto calculators. You can find an array of these online calculators online, but the ones from Ruled. Me and Perfect Keto are both good. There are also keto smartphone apps that not only include macronutrient calculators but also easy methods to track your calorie and macronutrient consumption over the day to make it easy to stick to your macros.

Speaking of tracking your macronutrient and calorie consumption, this is generally really important on the ketogenic diet. This is because it is much easier to consume twenty-five net carbs than you might think, and if you aren't tracking your carb intake, you are likely to double or more what you should be eating.

On the ketogenic diet, you can enjoy plenty of healthy fats, fish, seafood, meat, low-starch vegetables, berries, nuts, and seeds. But, to gain the most success, it is better to go into detail about the ingredients you shouldn't be eating. These ingredients can mess up your macronutrient ratio and throw off your nutrition.

FOODS TO AVOID

Grains

While grains may have their health benefits and be full of fiber, you can also get these nutrients elsewhere. The human diet does not require grain consumption. The truth is while grains may have some benefits, they are ridiculously high in both total and net carbohydrates, making them incompatible with the ketogenic diet. A single serving of brown rice contains a shocking forty-two net carbs, which is almost double your net carb intake for an entire day.

Although, some people do try what is known as the targeted ketogenic diet, which is a version of the diet specifically designed for those who complete extended and strenuous workouts. With the targeted ketogenic diet, a person will consume a small serving of a carb-heavy food, such as grains, thirty to forty minutes before working out.

Starchy Vegetables and Legumes

Some vegetables are high in carbohydrates. This includes potatoes, beans, beets, corn, and more. Yes, these vegetables may have nutritional benefits, but you can get these same nutrients in low-carb vegetable alternatives. To put into perspective how high in carbs these options can be, a medium-sized white potato contains forty-three net carbs (more than a serving of brown rice!), a standard sweet potato contains twenty-three net carbs, and a serving of black beans contains twenty-five net carbs.

Better Alternatives:

- Peppers
- Kale
- Radishes
- Cauliflower
- Green beans
- Asparagus
- Spinach
- Avocados
- Zucchini

- Tomatoes
- Celery
- Lettuce
- Swiss chard
- Cucumber
- Cabbage
- Broccoli
- Olives
- Mustard and turnip greens
- Squash

Sugary Fruits

Most fruits contain a high sugar content, meaning that they are also high in carbohydrates, will spike your blood sugar, and cause an insulin reaction. To avoid this, it is important to avoid most fruits. The exception is that you can enjoy berries, lemons, and limes in moderation. Some people will also enjoy a small serving of melon as a treat from time to time, but watch your portion size as it can add up quickly!

Milk and Low-Fat Dairy Products

As you can enjoy dairy products such as cheese on the ketogenic diet, you may consider trying milk. Sadly, milk is much higher in carbohydrates than cheese, with a glass of two-percent milk containing twelve carbs, half of your daily total. Instead, choose low-carb and dairy-free milk alternatives such as almond, coconut, and soy milk.

You may consider using low-fat cheeses instead of full fat to reduce the saturated fats you are consuming. But, if you are looking to reduce your saturated fat intake, choose lighter cuts of meat rather than low-fat dairy products. The reason for this is because when the cheese is made with low-fat dairy, it naturally has a higher carbohydrate content, which will cut into your daily net carb total.

Cashews, Pistachios, and Chestnuts

While you can enjoy nuts and seeds in moderation, keep in mind that nuts contain a moderate level of carbohydrates, and therefore should be eaten in moderation. However, some nuts are high in carbs and thus are not fed on the ketogenic diet, including cashews, pistachios, and chestnuts.

If you want to enjoy nuts, instead of these options, you can fully enjoy almonds, pecans, walnuts, macadamia nuts, and other options.

Most Natural Sweeteners

While you can certainly enjoy sugar-free natural sweeteners such as stevia, monk fruit, and sugar alcohols, you should avoid natural sweeteners that contain sugar. Suffice to say the sugar content makes these sweeteners naturally high in carbs. But, not only that, they will also spike your blood sugar and insulin. This means you should avoid things such as honey, agave, maple, coconut palm sugar, and dates.

Alcohol

Alcohol is not generally enjoyed on the ketogenic diet, as your body will be unable to burn off calories while your liver attempts to process alcohol. Many people also find that when they are in a state of ketosis, they get drunk more quickly and experience more severe hangovers. Not only that, but alcohol adds unnecessary calories and carbohydrates to your diet.

The worst offenders to choose would be margaritas, piña coladas, sangrias, Bloody Mary, whiskey sours, cosmopolitans, and regular beers.

But, if you do choose to drink alcohol regardless of drink in moderation and choose low-carb versions such as rum, vodka, tequila, whiskey, and gin. The next-best options would be dry wines and light beers.

Chapter Eight

HOW TO EXERCISE WHILE FASTING

Frequently, people are told to exercise and decrease calories when trying to lose weight. Simply take in fewer calories and expend more. But, losing weight is not this simple. After all, many people will try this method for years with little to no success in weight loss. That's because while this approach may seem rather simple, there is some important understanding many people are lacking. If you attempt to push yourself through dieting and intense exercise continuously, you will only deprive your body of essential nutrients and wear yourself out both physically and mentally.

Part of the problem that many people run into without realizing is a hormone imbalance. When a person decreases their food intake and increases their exercise in the wrong way, it will cause the hormones cortisol, leptin, and ghrelin to increase. When this happens, a person experiences increased hunger, increased weight retention, and added physical fatigue. Not only do all of these cause problems on their own, but it can also result in a person giving in to cravings and giving up on exercise.

Thankfully, intermittent fasting has been proven through study after study to be much more useful than dieting in weight loss. However, you can further increase weight loss by adding exercise to your routine, as well. In this chapter, you will learn how to pair exercise with intermittent fasting for optimal success, and without creating roadblocks, such as hemorrhage imbalances, that will impede your results.

You will be happy to know that the effects of exercise are increased when you are in a fasted state. This is because you will have few calories in your system. Therefore, your body will be forced to rely on burning off body fat for energy. Studies have repeatedly shown that when a person exercises in a fasted state, they burn off more body fat than they otherwise would. This means you can work out less and experience more weight loss! But, while the idea of increased weight loss may cause you to push yourself more to get the results you hope for sooner, it is important to take your time and listen to your body. If you push your body's limits too much, you can develop not only injuries but also hormonal imbalances and weakened health.

Most people who accomplish low to moderate intensity exercises will not experience diminished athletic performance. However, athletes and those who perform high-intensity exercise might notice a slight decrease in their performance, so they might want to participate in sporting activities during their eating window rather than their fasting window to increase energy.

The reason that athletes and those who practice high-intensity exercises may experience slight performance decreases during their fasting window is due to API energy. This source of energy is a result of glucose being stored within the muscles, which allows people to quickly react at high intensities. For instance, it is API energy that will fuel your body if you suddenly have to begin sprinting from danger. As the glucose for API energy is being stored in your muscles at all times, up to two-thousand calories worth at a time, your muscles can quickly jump to action without preparation. But, if you are in a fasting window without glucose being stored in your muscles, you will find that this energy source is lacking, thereby making short-term/high-intensity exercise more difficult. The result is that those who complete sports, bodybuilding, and CrossFit will be affected.

While you can perform high-intensity exercises while in a fasted state, you must do it while carefully listening to your body, and if you find that you become overly weak, dizzy, or light-headed, then it is important that you either reduce your pace or take a short break before resuming your workout.

You are less likely to notice this decrease in energy if you are only a few hours into your fasting window, but if you are twelve hours or more into a fast, then you are more likely to experience this performance decrease. Therefore, if you do want to practice a high-intensity workout during your fast, try to schedule it earlier in your fasting window rather than later.

If you are not on the ketogenic diet, then it can be a good idea to increase your healthy carbohydrate intake before beginning your fasting window if you plan to exercise. Simply eating some brown rice or starchy vegetables can help you to increase your ATP energy supply, helping you later in the day during your workout.

Thankfully, studies on short-term fasting and exercise have found that as a person adjusts to both fasting and working out, it becomes easier. Over time, your body will adapt to the decreased ATP energy and be able to perform better even when in a fasted state.

The good news for people who don't care for intense exercise is that moderate cardio is the ideal workout for a fasted state. This is because cardio does not use API energy, meaning that you will be able to complete it at full performance without any problems. Many types of exercises can be achieved with cardio, and the weight loss effects of all of them will be increased when you are in a fasted state. This can be especially helpful for women as they age, as cardio improves both heart and lung health.

If you are on the ketogenic diet, then you will be happy to know that cardio doesn't require you to consume a larger quantity of carbohydrates, as it doesn't utilize API energy. You can maintain your state of ketosis and promote weight loss simultaneously. Cardio is especially perfect for completing during your fasting window, as you never want to achieve a cardio workout on a full stomach. While some people may mistakenly eat directly before a cardio workout, this is damaging as the blood flow to your muscles will interfere with your digestive system. When this happens, it can not only cause digestive distress, but it also prevents your body from absorbing the nutrients from your meal. If you are going to be workout out, only do so after fasting for three to four hours minimum.

While many people have been advised by trainers or workout enthusiasts to eat a lot of protein directly before their workout, often in the form of a protein shake or smoothie, new scientific research found that this is not needed. Not only is it doing your body a disservice to eat directly before working out, but studies have found that it does not improve your workout at all. It doesn't even improve bodybuilding, as you can increase muscle growth as long as you eat protein within a few hours of weightlifting.

How you eat and fast can also affect your insulin sensitivity, which is important as reduced insulin sensitivity is a part of and precursor to type II diabetes, which many women develop as they age. In one study, athletes and bodybuilders completed a variety of fasting and eating methods to compare their insulin sensitivity. One group consumed a carb-heavy meal directly before their workout, one trained while in a fasted state, and the control group did not work out at all. All three groups consumed the same meals, and the only thing that varied was when they ate in relation to their workout. The study revealed that while the first and second group ate the same foods and the same amount of food, the group that exercised while in a fasted state experienced improved insulin sensitivity. Not only that, but this group also was able to tolerate glucose better.

The human growth hormone, also known as HGH, experienced increased production when you are in a fasted state. This is good news, as it can help you increase muscle strength and mass while workout out. Even if you are not looking to increase overall muscle mass, we can all benefit from strengthening muscles, especially as they begin to weaken as we age. You can keep your muscles stronger and younger as you age if you practice exercise in a fasted state, at a much more effective rate than if you exercised without fasting. This is important, as when muscles become weakened and aged a person experiences an increased risk of energy, they are more likely to fall, and the body overall begins to run less efficiently.

Pairing exercise and fasting can create antioxidants that reduce fatigue, increase healing, produce more energy, and improve overall health as you age. As you are most likely well aware of, antioxidants are vital for reducing cellular aging and decay. Not only will this protect your muscle health, but overall body health, even the health of your brain.

There are a few things you should keep in mind while working out during a fasted state to get the most out of your workout while saving your energy and maintaining your health. Thankfully, you working out in a fasted state is much easier than you might think, and you will find it much more effective than exercise alone. First, it is often easiest for most people to practice a moderate-range fast of fourteen or sixteen hours, skipping breakfast and making lunch the first meal of the day. If you are doing this, then you can easily workout first thing in the morning when you are a decent way into your fast, and it will be the most productive. You will feel more energy at this time as you are well-rested, and then you can recharge at lunchtime with your meal breaking your fast.

When exercising in this way, your body in a fasted state will activate the sympathetic nervous system, therefore allowing you to burn more fat and lose more weight. But it is important to remember that just because you are fasting doesn't mean you need water any less. It is even more important to stay hydrated. Be sure that while you are exercising, you drink plenty of water and that during your eating window, you consume plenty of electrolytes. Although, you can also purchase zero-calorie sugar-free sports drinks that are naturally sweetened with stevia leaf, and you can enjoy these during even a fasted workout.

When you are exercising, listen to your body and use common sense to know your limits. These limits will vary for everyone based on their exact age, fitness level, health, how long they have been in a fasted state, whether or not they are taking medicine, and more. Only you and your doctor can determine exactly where your limit is, and to avoid pushing past this limit. It is important to listen to all the signs and signals your body is giving you.

If you find that you struggle to exercise after long periods of fasting, then instead do your workout only a few hours into your fast rather than near the end of it. You might find that certain types of exercise are easier for you to complete in a fasted state than others. Or, you might find that there is a specific amount of time after your workout that you feel best eating at. For instance, while one person may be able to wait hours after their workout to eat, another person may only be able to wait thirty to sixty minutes.

Listen to your body and plan your meals, fasting, and exercise routine accordingly.

Chapter Nine

RECIPES

While you can consume any diet while practicing intermittent fasting, you must consume nutritious and healthy foods if you hope to benefit your health. In this chapter, we will share some of our favorite recipes that are full of nutrients necessary in a healthy lifestyle. Some of these recipes will be low-carb/ketogenic, whereas others, so that both individuals who choose to pair the ketogenic diet with fasting and those that do not can equally experience benefits from these recipes.

BREAKFAST

These recipes are the perfect breakfast. Whether you are enjoying breakfast at 7 am or noon, it doesn't matter. You will find that these recipes are not only full of delicious flavor that will bring you back for more time, and again, they are also full of nutrition that will keep you satisfied and healthy.

SWEET POTATO AND CHICKPEA HASH

This hash is simple to cook, but full of flavor and crispy! Not only that, but it is also vegan! Enjoy it served as-is, or you can enjoy it with either freshly sliced avocado or a fried egg for added flavor and nutrition. With this hash, you will stay full and satisfied all day long.

Details:

Number of Servings: **4**

Time Needed to Prepare: 10 minutes
Time Required to Cook: 45 minutes
Total Preparation/Cook Time: 55 minutes

Number of Calories in Individual Servings: 343
Protein Grams: 12
Fat Grams: 17
Total Carbohydrates Grams: 40
Net Carbohydrates Grams: 25

Ingredients:

- Sweet potatoes, cut into 3/4-inch cubes – 1.5 pounds
- Chickpeas, canned, drained and rinsed – 15 ounces
- Bell pepper, red or orange, diced – 1
- Bell pepper, green, diced – 1
- Onion, medium, diced – 1
- Garlic powder – 1 teaspoon
- Sea salt – 1.5 teaspoons

- Olive oil – 2 tablespoons
- Black pepper, ground - .25 teaspoons
- Tahini paste – 4 tablespoons
- Water – 4 tablespoons
- Sea salt - .5 teaspoon
- Lemon juice – 2 tablespoons
- Sriracha sauce – 2 tablespoons

Instructions:

Begin by setting your oven to a temperature of Fahrenheit four-hundred and twenty-five degrees. Then, line a large aluminum baking sheet with either kitchen parchment or a silicone mat.

Place the diced onion, sweet potatoes, and bell peppers on the prepared baking sheet, along with the rinsed chickpeas. Drizzle the olive oil, black ground pepper, garlic powder, and 1.5 teaspoons of sea salt over the vegetables and then toss them all together until the vegetables are well coated in the oil and seasoning.

Spread the vegetable mixture out evenly on the pan so that the sweet potatoes, beans, peppers, and onions are all in a single layer. This will allow the hash to cook consistently and become crispy.

Place the sheet of vegetables in the center of your oven and let it cook for twenty-five minutes, stirring the vegetables once halfway through the cooking time.

Increase the temperature of your oven to Fahrenheit five-hundred degrees, stir the vegetables again, and cook for an additional twenty minutes. Once again, halfway through the cooking time, stir the vegetables.

While the vegetables cook whisk together the tahini paste, water, sriracha sauce, lemon juice, and remaining sea salt.

Once the hash is finished cooking, serve it with the sriracha tahini sauce, and enjoy. Optionally, you can add avocado slices or a fried egg on the side.

OATMEAL PANCAKES

The bananas and oats pair beautifully for a sweet and nutty flavor, but they also add extra value to these pancakes. Rather than making traditional pancakes that contain only refined sugar and flours, you can gain the fiber and nutrients from both the oats and the bananas. These nutrients will keep you healthy and full.

Details:

Number of Servings: **5**

Time Needed to Prepare: 3 minutes
Time Required to Cook: 10 minutes
Total Preparation/Cook Time: 13 minutes

Number of Calories in Individual Servings: 362
Protein Grams: 14
Fat Grams: 6
Total Carbohydrates Grams: 65
Net Carbohydrates Grams: 56

Ingredients:

- Bananas, ripe, large – 2
- Rolled oats – 2.25 cups
- Coconut milk – 1 cup
- Egg – 1
- Maple syrup – 1 tablespoon
- Baking powder – 1.5 teaspoons
- Sea salt - .25 teaspoon
- Cinnamon, ground - .5 teaspoon

- Vanilla extract – 1 teaspoon
- Butter for cooking

Instructions:

Place all of the ingredients, except for the butter, in a blender. Blend on high speed until the oats and bananas have broken down, about one to two minutes.

Heat a large electric griddle or a non-stick skillet over medium-low heat.

Once the griddle or skillet is preheated, add a little of the butter and coat the pan with it. Then, using a small ladle, pour small scoops onto the griddle, with each pancake holding about .25 cups of batter.

Cook the pancakes for two to three minutes before flipping and cooking a couple more minutes.

Serve the pancakes with sliced bananas and maple syrup.

KETO BURRITO WRAP WITH BACON AND AVOCADO

These keto burritos are low in carbs and high in important healthy fats, such as those from avocados. Whether you are on the ketogenic diet or not, you will find that these breakfast burritos are delicious and a great way to start your day! The fats and protein within these burritos will keep you energized and satisfied for hours to come.

Details:

Number of Servings: **2**

Number of Calories in Individual Servings: 426
Protein Grams: 13
Fat Grams: 39
Total Carbohydrates Grams: 6
Net Carbohydrates Grams: 2

Ingredients:

- Eggs – 2
- Bacon, cooked – 4 slices
- Half n' half – 2 tablespoons
- Sea salt - .25 teaspoon
- Black pepper, ground - .125 teaspoon
- Mayonnaise – 2 tablespoons
- Butter – 2 tablespoons
- Roma tomato, sliced – 1
- Romaine lettuce, chopped – 1 cup

- Avocado, sliced - .5

Instructions:

Vigorously whisk together the eggs with the sea salt, black ground pepper, and half n' half until the egg white proteins break down and combine thoroughly with the egg yolk.

In a non-stick skillet over a preheated temperature of medium heat, melt half of the butter. Once the butter has melted, add in half of the egg mixture. Tilt the pan around to ensure the egg covers the entire surface evenly.

Cover the pan with a lid and allow the egg to cook for a minute until set. Once the bottom of the egg is cooked and can move around the pan gently flip it over to cook the other side the rest of the way.

Once both sides of the egg are cooked gently, remove it from the pan and allow it to rest on a plate with a paper towel, allowing it to remove any excess oil.

Melt the remaining butter in the pan and cook the other half of the egg in the same manner.

Once both egg crepes are cooked, spread your mayonnaise over one side of each of them, add on the lettuce, tomato, avocado, and bacon. Roll them up like a burrito and enjoy!

KETO BLUEBERRY PANCAKES

These low-carb pancakes will remind you of all your favorite classic blueberry pancakes, but without the guilt! To keep these low-carb, you can enjoy them with fresh berries and whipped cream or Lakanto brand sugar-free maple-flavored syrup. These options are much lower in carbs than traditional maple syrup but just as delicious!

Details:

Number of Servings: **3**

Time Needed to Prepare: 3 minutes
Time Required to Cook: 10 minutes
Total Preparation/Cook Time: 13 minutes

Number of Calories in Individual Servings: 363
Protein Grams: 14
Fat Grams: 28
Total Carbohydrates Grams: 17
Net Carbohydrates Grams: 11

Ingredients:

- Eggs – 4
- Almond flour – 1.33 cup
- Almond milk – 3 tablespoons
- Vanilla extract - .5 teaspoon
- Baking powder – 2 teaspoons
- Sea salt - .25 teaspoon
- Swerve sugar-free sweetener – 1 tablespoon

- Blueberries - .75 cup
- Butter – 2 tablespoons

Instructions:

In a bowl, whisk together your eggs before adding in the almond flour, almond milk, vanilla extract, baking powder, and Swerve sweetener.

Once the batter is fully combined, gently fold in the blueberries, either fresh or frozen.

Heat a large electric griddle or a non-stick skillet over medium heat. Once hot, grease the skillet with the reserved butter and ladle the pancakes onto the pan. Each pancake should contain about .25 cups of batter.

Once the first side of the pancakes is cooked and golden, gently flip them over. Be careful not to mess with the pancakes while they are cooking. You only want to touch them when flipping.

Once both sides of the pancakes are cooked, remove them from the stove and serve them with fruit and whipped cream or Lakanto's sugar-free maple-flavored syrup.

KETO SAUSAGE AND CHEESE VEGETABLE FRITTATA

This frittata is full of breakfast sausage, vegetables, cream cheese, and cheddar cheese. You will love every slice of this delectable frittata, and even more than that, you will like how it gives you a week's worth of breakfast to store in the fridge or freezer to effortlessly enjoy.

Details:

Number of Servings: **8**

Time Needed to Prepare: 10 minutes
Time Required to Cook: 50 minutes
Total Preparation/Cook Time: 1 hour

Number of Calories in Individual Servings: 389
Protein Grams: 20
Fat Grams: 31
Total Carbohydrates Grams: 5
Net Carbohydrates Grams: 4

Ingredients:

- Eggs – 6
- Cream cheese, cut into cubes – 8 ounces
- Ground breakfast sausage – 1 pound
- Cheddar cheese, shredded – 8 ounces
- Kale, chopped – 1.5 cups
- Onion, small, diced – 1
- Bell pepper, diced – 1

- Garlic, minced – 3 cloves
- Half n' half - .5 cup
- Water - .5 cup

Instructions:

Preheat your oven to a temperature of Fahrenheit three-hundred and seventy-five degrees.

In a large skillet, which should be set to medium-high heat, add the breakfast sausage, onion, garlic, and bell pepper, and cook it until the sausage is browned all the way through. Drain off any excess fat after cooking.

Add the cream cheese to the skillet and stir it into the meat until it is fully melted. Place the chopped kale into the skillet, cover it with a lid, and then allow it to cook for an additional two minutes until it has reduced in size.

In a bowl, vigorously whisk together the eggs, half n' half, and water until the egg white proteins are fully broken down into the yolk and liquid.

Grease an eleven by seven-inch casserole dish and then add the sausage and vegetable mixture into it. Sprinkle the cheddar cheese over the top before pouring the egg mixture over everything.

Use a spoon to slightly move the ingredients around so the eggs get between all the vegetables and meat.

Place the casserole dish in the oven and allow it to cook until the center of the frittata is fully cooked for about forty minutes. Remove the dish from the oven and allow it to cool for ten minutes before serving.

KETO CHEESE AND SAUSAGE SCONES

These scones are a fantastic way to enjoy the morning, whether you are relaxing at the dining room table or rushing out on the town. They are full of delicious cheddar cheese, breakfast sausage, sweet peppers, and onion for amazing flavor.

Details:

Number of Servings: **4**

Time Needed to Prepare: 5 minutes
Time Required to Cook: 10 minutes
Total Preparation/Cook Time: 15 minutes

Number of Calories in Individual Servings: 307
Protein Grams: 18
Fat Grams: 23
Total Carbohydrates Grams: 7
Net Carbohydrates Grams: 4

Ingredients:

- Eggs – 3
- Cheddar cheese, shredded – 1 cup
- Ground breakfast sausage – 4 ounces
- Almond flour - .75 cup
- Onion, diced - .5 cup
- Bell pepper, diced - .5 cup
- Sea salt - .5 teaspoon
- Black pepper, ground - .5 teaspoon

Instructions:

Preheat your oven to a temperature of Fahrenheit three-hundred and seventy-five degrees and prepare an aluminum baking sheet by lining it with either kitchen parchment or a silicone liner.

Place the breakfast sausage, bell pepper, and onion in a skillet and cook it all together over medium heat until the meat is cooked all the way through and the vegetables are soft. Remove it from the heat and allow it to cool.

In a bowl, mix the almond flour, black pepper, baking powder, and sea salt.

Into another bowl, combine the eggs and the cheese. Add this mixture to the almond flour mixture along with the cooled vegetables and sausage. Combine fully.

Using a large spoon, scoop out the dough into portions, with each scone containing about two tablespoons of dough. The mixture will be sticky, but place it on the pan the best as you can. Each dough portion should be placed about two inches apart. Slightly flatten the dough mounds with your fingers.

Place the scones in the oven until cooked all the way through and golden, about eight to ten minutes. Once done, allow the scones to cool for a few minutes before enjoying.

LUNCH

These simple meals are the perfect way to enjoy an afternoon. Whether you are at home, work, or on the go, you will find simple go-to solutions to eat healthy and delicious meals. You will find both meals that you can prepare ahead of time and store in the fridge to enjoy throughout the week and quick and simple meals to prepare at a moment's notice.

SHRIMP GREEK SALAD

This salad is satisfying and delicious, and it will keep you full and nourished all day long! Whether you are preparing to start your fast or break a fast, you will find that this is the perfect meal. With the fibrous brown rice, fresh vegetables, and refreshing shrimp, you will find this salad different from any other.

Details:

Number of Servings: **5**

Time Needed to Prepare: 10 minutes
Time Required to Cook: 0 minutes
Total Preparation/Cook Time: 10 minutes

Number of Calories in Individual Servings: 500
Protein Grams: 22
Fat Grams: 25
Total Carbohydrates Grams: 46
Net Carbohydrates Grams: 41

Ingredients:

- Brown rice, cooked – 4 cups
- Shrimp, medium, cooked – 1 pound
- Cucumber, diced – 1
- Roma tomatoes, diced – 2
- Parsley, chopped - .75 cup
- Scallions, thinly sliced – 3
- Kalamata olives pitted and chopped - .5 cup
- Feta cheese, crumbled – 6 ounces

- Olive oil - .33 cup
- Garlic, minced – 3 cloves
- Lemon juice – .33 cup
- Oregano, dried – 2 teaspoons
- Sea salt – 1 teaspoon

Instructions:

Add the cooked brown rice, shrimp, and vegetables together in a large salad bowl and toss them together.

In a smaller bowl, vigorously whisk together the olive oil, lemon juice, garlic, oregano, and sea salt until fully combined.

Pour the prepared vinaigrette over the tossed salad and once again toss to fully coat the salad in the vinaigrette. Carefully fold in the feta cheese to prevent it from falling apart.

Store the salad in the fridge for up to three to four days.

SWEET PEPPER NACHOS

Rather than fattening chips, these nachos are made with low-carb sweet bell peppers. You will love the bell peppers filled with taco-flavored beef, cheddar cheese, fresh tomatoes, cilantro, and sour cream. Of course, you can also add in any of your favorite nacho toppings to customize these to perfection.

The Details:

Number of Servings: **5**

Time Needed to Prepare: 10 minutes
Time Required to Cook: 15 minutes
Total Preparation/Cook Time: 25 minutes

Number of Calories in Individual Servings: 410
Protein Grams: 23
Fat Grams: 30
Total Carbohydrates Grams: 10
Net Carbohydrates Grams: 8

Ingredients:

- Bell peppers – 3
- Ground beef, 80/20 – 1 pound
- Cheddar cheese, shredded – 1 cup
- Chili powder – 1 teaspoon
- Sea salt – 1 teaspoon
- Onion powder - .5 teaspoon
- Cumin – 1 teaspoon
- Black pepper, ground - .5 teaspoon

- Garlic powder – .5 teaspoon
- Roma tomatoes, diced – 2
- Sour cream - .5 cup
- Cilantro, chopped - .5 cup

Instructions:

Slice around the top of the bell peppers so that you can cleanly remove the stems. Once the stems are removed, pull out the seeds and membrane. Slice each of the bell peppers into six portions that are shaped like boats or chips. Set the bell peppers aside.

Place the ground beef in a large skillet and cook it until it is fully cooked through. Drain off any excess fat and then stir in the diced tomatoes, chopped cilantro, chili powder, cumin, sea salt, black pepper, onion powder, and garlic powder.

Preheat the oven to a temperature of Fahrenheit three-hundred and seventy-five degrees and line an aluminum baking pan with either a silicone mat or kitchen parchment.

Place the bell pepper boats on the baking sheet and then fill them with the beef mixture. Top the beef off with the shredded cheese. Cook the bell pepper boats in the oven until hot and the cheese is melted about ten minutes.

Once the peppers are done cooking, top them with the sour cream and enjoy!

Optional: if you would like the bell peppers to be softer, you can place them in a glass baking dish with a few tablespoons of water, cover the dish with aluminum foil, and allow it to cook in the oven for fifteen minutes.

SPAGHETTI SQUASH GARLIC NOODLES WITH CHICKEN

These noodles are perfect for enjoying on-the-go, as they can be eaten either hot or cold. Simply pack up your noodles in a warm thermos or a cold bag with some ice, and you have a full nutritious meal ready to go. This means that even if you need to break your fast during the middle of your workday or while running errands, you will be prepared with a tasty and nutritious meal with little effort.

Details:

Number of Servings: **4**

Time Needed to Prepare: 10 minutes
Time Required to Cook: 25 minutes
Total Preparation/Cook Time: 35 minutes

Number of Calories in Individual Servings: 438

Protein Grams: 33
Fat Grams: 14
Total Carbohydrates Grams: 49
Net Carbohydrates Grams: 38

Ingredients:

- Spaghetti squash, 5 pounds, cooked – 1
- Zucchini, julienned – 1
- Red bell pepper, small, minced – 1
- Cilantro, chopped - .5 cup
- Almonds, toasted, chopped - .25 cup

- Soy sauce or coconut aminos replacement - .66 cup
- Coconut milk, full fat - .25 cup
- Garlic, minced – 6 cloves
- Ginger, grated – 2 tablespoons
- Red curry paste – 2 tablespoons
- Fish sauce or vegan replacement – 2 tablespoons
- Lakanto golden sugar-free monk fruit sweetener – 3 tablespoons
- Chicken thighs, chopped into 1-inch cubes – 1 pound

Instructions:

If your spaghetti squash is not already cooked, you can prepare it by chopping it in half lengthwise, removing the seeds, and then placing it facing upward on a baking sheet. Lightly brush the squash with oil and then cook it until tender (about twenty-five minutes) at a temperature of Fahrenheit four-hundred and fifty degrees.

Prepare the chicken by placing it in a large non-stick skillet over a temperature of medium-high heat and allow it to cook until fully cooked through about seven to nine minutes. The internal temperature of the chicken must reach one-hundred and sixty-five degrees Fahrenheit to avoid food poisoning. Set aside.

In a blender, combine the soy sauce, coconut milk, garlic, ginger, red curry paste, fish sauce, and Lakanto sweetener until no chunks are remaining.

Run a fork through the hot spaghetti squash to form noodles out of the flesh. Transfer the "noodles" to a large bowl and toss them together with the cooked chicken, blended sauce, cilantro, zucchini, red bell pepper, and almonds.

Serve the noodles hot or cold. Store in the fridge for five to six days.

KETO CALIFORNIA ROLL BOWLS

Even if you are eating a low-carb/keto diet, you can still enjoy your favorite California rolls with these delicious bowls! They are full of protein from the crab, along with other important nutrients from the cauliflower rice, avocado, cucumber, nori, and sesame seeds. Your favorite food is now healthier than ever!

Details:

Number of Servings: **2**

Number of Calories in Individual Servings: 310
Protein Grams: 19
Fat Grams: 20
Total Carbohydrates Grams: 13
Net Carbohydrates Grams: 6

Ingredients:

- Cauliflower rice – 1.5 cups
- Avocado, thinly sliced - .5
- Cucumber, thinly sliced – 1
- Scallions, thinly sliced – 1
- Nori sheet, cut into small pieces - .5
- Crabmeat, canned – 6 ounces
- Seasoned rice vinegar – 1 tablespoon
- White sesame seeds, toasted - .5 tablespoon
- Black sesame seeds, toasted - .5 tablespoon
- Mayonnaise – 2 tablespoons
- Sriracha sauce – 2 teaspoons

Instructions:

In a bowl, whisk together the sriracha sauce and mayonnaise until they are fully combined and then set aside.

Steam the cauliflower rice in the microwave or on the stove until it is tender. Once done cooking, stir in the rice vinegar.

Divide the cooked cauliflower rice between two bowls and top it with the cucumbers, avocado, scallions, and crab meat. Drizzle the sriracha mayonnaise over the top and then sprinkle on the sesame seeds.

Enjoy the bowls immediately or store them in the fridge for up to three days before enjoying. Wait to add the chopped nori until immediately before serving so that it remains crispy.

KETO CHICKEN AVOCADO SALAD

This chicken salad is one of the most flavorful you will ever taste, with mashed avocado and Ranch dressing in place of mayonnaise, and with added bacon and cheddar cheese. This chicken salad can be served with your favorite low-carb snacking options or butterhead lettuce, as used in the recipe.

Details:

Number of Servings: **4**

Time Needed to Prepare: 5 minutes
Time Required to Cook: 0 minutes
Total Preparation/Cook Time: 5 minutes

Number of Calories in Individual Servings: 434
Protein Grams: 32
Fat Grams: 29
Total Carbohydrates Grams: 9
Net Carbohydrates Grams: 4

Ingredients:

- Chicken, cooked, diced – 2 cups
- Avocado, lightly mashed – 1
- Bacon, cooked, chopped – 6 slices
- Sea salt – 1 teaspoon
- Cheddar cheese, shredded - .75 cup
- Celery, diced - .75 cup
- Scallions, thinly sliced - .75 cup
- Primal Kitchen's Ranch or Caesar dressing - .25 cup

- Black pepper, ground - .25 teaspoon
- Butter lettuce – 2 heads

Instructions:

In a large bowl, toss together all ingredients, except the lettuce, until fully combined and coated in the dressing. Taste and adjust the seasonings to taste, add more dressing if desired.

Serve immediately with the butter lettuce or save in the fridge for up to five days.

DINNER

Whether you are craving your favorite comfort food or a full meal that you can share with the whole family, you will love these healthy and delicious dinners that are perfect for enjoying before beginning an overnight fast.

BIG MAC SALAD BOWL

No matter how delicious and nutritious food might be, we all have our guilty pleasures. One of these comfort foods for many people is the Big Mac burger. However, you can allow yourself to enjoy all the flavors of this favorite meal without the fattening ingredients that will leave you feeling bloated and sluggish. This version of the Big Mac is full of all your favorite ingredients but without the unhealthy additives. You can enjoy this low-carb/keto Big Mac, while still gaining health and losing weight.

While it may be typical to use full-fat meats on the ketogenic diet, in this recipe, you want to use lean ground beef. Otherwise, the burger will be overly greasy. Trust me; it's perfect this way.

Details:

Number of Servings: **4**

Time Needed to Prepare: 7 minutes
Time Required to Cook: 7 minutes
Total Preparation/Cook Time: 14 minutes

Number of Calories in Individual Servings: 525
Protein Grams: 30
Fat Grams: 41
Total Carbohydrates Grams: 5
Net Carbohydrates Grams: 4

Ingredients:

- Ground beef, lean – 1 pound

- Black pepper, ground – 1 teaspoon
- Onion, sliced in rounds - .5 cup
- Cheddar cheese, shredded – 1 cup
- Sea salt – 1 teaspoon
- Pickles, sliced - .25 cup
- Iceberg lettuce, chopped – 4 cups
- Yellow mustard – 4 teaspoons
- Mayonnaise - .5 cup
- Vinegar – 2 teaspoons
- Lakanto monk fruit sweetener – 1.5 teaspoons
- Pickles, diced – 4 teaspoons
- Onion, finely minced – 1 tablespoon
- Paprika, smoked - .25 teaspoon

Instructions:

Begin by making your special sauce. To do this, whisk together the mustard, mayonnaise, vinegar, sweetener, diced pickles, minced onion, and smoked paprika. Set the sauce aside to allow the flavors to meld together. The sauce can be made up to a week in advance, and it tastes even better after resting overnight in the fridge.

Heat a large skillet over a temperature of medium heat and brown the ground beef. Once it is mostly cooked with only a little pink remaining add in the sea salt and black pepper, and then finish cooking it until the pink disappears, and it is cooked all the way through.

Divide the lettuce, pickles, onions, and cheese evenly between four bowls, and then add the browned beef on top. By placing the hot beef on top of the other ingredients, you will melt the cheese.

Drizzle the special sauce over the top of the Big Mac bowls and serve immediately.

"STUFFED" CABBAGE CASSEROLE

This low-carb "stuffed" cabbage casserole is much easier to make than traditional stuffed cabbage, as you simply layer everything in the pan and allow the flavors to meld together.

Details:

Number of Servings: **5**

Time Needed to Prepare: 5 minutes
Time Required to Cook: 25 minutes
Total Preparation/Cook Time: 30 minutes

Number of Calories in Individual Servings: 398
Protein Grams: 26
Fat Grams: 24
Total Carbohydrates Grams: 20
Net Carbohydrates Grams: 14

Ingredients:

- Ground beef, 85/15 – 1 pound
- Olive oil – 1 tablespoon
- Bell pepper, orange, sliced – 1
- Sweet onion, sliced – 1
- Garlic, minced – 3 cloves
- Diced tomatoes – 1 can
- Sea salt – 1 teaspoon
- Smoked paprika - .5 teaspoon
- Garlic powder - .5 teaspoon
- Dried oregano – .5 teaspoon

- Onion powder - .5 teaspoon
- Black pepper, ground - .5 teaspoon
- Green cabbage, chopped – 1 head
- Cheddar cheese, shredded – 1 cup

Instructions:

To a large skillet over medium-high heat, add the olive oil, ground beef, bell pepper, and onion. Allow the vegetables and meat to cook together until the beef is mostly browned. Add in the garlic and cook until the meat is fully cooked.

Into the skillet, add the canned tomatoes and seasonings, stirring the ingredients all together. Add the cabbage to the top of the skillet, cover the skillet with a lid, and cook until the cabbage is tender about fifteen minutes.

Sprinkle the cheese over the top of the dish and place the lid back on top for a couple of minutes, until the cheese is melted. Serve immediately and store any leftovers in the fridge for up to five or six days.

KETO CHILI

This low-carb chili is full of flavor and seasoning, complete with a touch of cocoa powder to deepen and meld the flavors together. Not only can you cook this chili on the stove for a quick meal, you can also cook it in a slow cooker for even deeper flavors, and an easy meal prepared ahead of time.

Details:

Number of Servings: **8**

Time Needed to Prepare: 5 minutes
Time Required to Cook: 40 minutes
Total Preparation/Cook Time: 45 minutes

Number of Calories in Individual Servings: 307
Protein Grams: 25
Fat Grams: 18
Total Carbohydrates Grams: 12
Net Carbohydrates Grams: 9

Ingredients:

- Ground beef, 85/15 – 2 pounds
- Jalapeno, seeds removed and diced – 1
- Bell pepper, diced – 1
- Beef broth – 32 ounces
- Tomato sauce – 15 ounces
- Tomatoes with green chilies – 10 ounces

- Tomato paste – 7 ounces
- Sea salt – 2 teaspoons
- Garlic, minced – 4 cloves
- Chili powder – 2 tablespoons
- Cocoa powder – 2 teaspoons
- Garlic powder – 1 teaspoon
- Cumin – 1 teaspoon
- Oregano, dried – 1 teaspoon
- Black pepper, ground - .5 teaspoon

Instructions:

In a large Dutch oven or pot brown the ground beef. Once fully cooked, drain off any excess fat.

Add the remaining ingredients and stir them all together until fully combined. Simmer the chili over low heat for thirty minutes, until the sauce has thickened and reduced. Serve immediately or store in the fridge for up to a week.

Alternatively, after browning the beef, you can combine all the ingredients in a slow cooker and then allow it to cook on low for four hours or high for two hours.

CREAMY ARTICHOKE SPINACH SOUP

This creamy soup is just like your favorite artichoke and spinach dip but without the guilt! You can now enjoy it low-carb for a complete meal, and any occasion!

Details:

Number of Servings: **6**

Time Needed to Prepare: 5 minutes
Time Required to Cook: 22 minutes
Total Preparation/Cook Time: 27 minutes

Number of Calories in Individual Servings: 440
Protein Grams: 12
Fat Grams: 37
Total Carbohydrates Grams: 17
Net Carbohydrates Grams: 12

Ingredients:

- Frozen Spinach, chopped – 9 ounces
- Artichoke hearts, canned and drained, chopped – 14 ounces
- Chicken broth – 4 cups
- Heavy cream – 1 cup
- Cream cheese – 8 ounces
- Parmesan cheese, grated – 1 cup
- Garlic, minced – 4 cloves
- Sea salt – 1 teaspoon
- Onion, diced – 1

- Butter – 2 tablespoons
- Black pepper, ground - .5 teaspoon

Instructions:

In a large Dutch oven or pot, melt the butter and then add in the onion, cooking it until slightly softened about five minutes. Add in the garlic and cook for one to two more minutes.

Add the spinach to the Dutch oven and allow it to thaw and cook until warmed through, about five to seven minutes, and then stir in the sea salt and black pepper.

Add the artichoke hearts and chicken broth to the pot and then allow it to heat about five to ten additional minutes.

Reduce the heat to low before adding in the cream cheese and heavy cream. Melt the cream cheese slowly, being careful not to curdle the cream. Stir in the Parmesan cheese.

Serve the soup immediately or store it in the fridge for up to six days.

DESSERT

KETO CHOCOLATE MOUSSE

This chocolate mousse only takes a few minutes to whip up and can be enjoyed immediately. Serve it as-is or pour it into a low-carb keto pie crust for a chocolate mousse pie.

Details:

Number of Servings: **4**

Time Needed to Prepare: 5 minutes
Time Required to Cook: 0 minutes
Total Preparation/Cook Time: 5 minutes

Number of Calories in Individual Servings: 324

Protein Grams: 3
Fat Grams: 34
Total Carbohydrates Grams: 6
Net Carbohydrates Grams: 4

Ingredients:

- Cocoa powder – .33 cup
- Lakanto monk fruit sweetener – 2 tablespoons
- Heavy whipping cream – 1.5 cups

Instructions:

Place the heavy cream in a bowl and use a hand mixer or stand mixer to beat it on medium speed.

Once the cream begins to thicken, add the monk fruit sweetener and cocoa and continue to beat it until stiff peaks form.

Serve the mousse immediately or store it in the fridge for up to twenty-four hours before enjoying it. If desired, you can serve it with Lily's stevia-sweetened chocolate for chunks.

NO-BAKE PEANUT BUTTER PIE

This pie is the perfect treat to serve at the holidays, at a potluck, or any other time you might be craving a sweet treat. No matter the occasion, you will find that this creamy no-bake peanut butter pie will offer you all the sweetness and flavor you are craving. If you want, you can even drizzle melted Lily's stevia-sweetened chocolate over the top.

Details:

Number of Servings: **8**

Time Needed to Prepare: 15 minutes
Time Required to Cook: 0 minutes
Total Preparation/Cook Time: 15 minutes

Number of Calories in Individual Servings: 518
Protein Grams: 12
Fat Grams: 49
Total Carbohydrates Grams: 12
Net Carbohydrates Grams: 9

Ingredients:

- Almond flour – 1 cup
- Butter softened – 2 tablespoons
- Vanilla - .5 teaspoon
- Lakanto monk fruit sweetener – 1.5 tablespoons
- Cocoa powder – 3 tablespoons
- Cream cheese softened – 16 ounces
- Heavy cream – .75 cup

- Vanilla – 2 teaspoons
- Swerve confectioner's sweetener - .66 cup
- Peanut butter or Sun Butter, unsweetened – .75 cup

Instructions:

Combine the almond flour, butter, .5 teaspoon of vanilla, Lakanto sweetener, and cocoa powder in a bowl with a fork until it forms a crumbly mixture. Press this mixture into a nine-inch pie plate and then allow it to chill in the fridge while you prepare the filling.

In a large bowl, beat together the cream cheese, peanut butter, confectioners Swerve, and remaining vanilla until light and creamy. Using a spatula scrape down the sides of the bowl before adding in the heavy cream.

Beat the filling some more until the heavy cream is incorporated and the mixture is once again light and creamy.

Pour the filling into the prepared crust and allow it to chill for two hours before serving. Slice and enjoy.

BERRIES WITH RICOTTA CREAM

This dessert is simple and quick to make with healthy fresh ingredients, making it the perfect treat year-round. However, it is especially delicious in the spring, when berries are in season.

Details:

Number of Servings: **4**

Time Needed to Prepare: 5 minutes
Time Required to Cook: 0 minutes
Total Preparation/Cook Time: 5 minutes

Number of Calories in Individual Servings: 217

Protein Grams: 11
Fat Grams: 15
Total Carbohydrates Grams: 9
Net Carbohydrates Grams: 7

Ingredients:

- Ricotta, whole milk – 1.5 cups
- Heavy cream – 2 tablespoons
- Lemon zest – 1.5 teaspoons
- Swerve confectioner's sweetener – .25 cup
- Vanilla extract – 1 teaspoon
- Blackberries - .5 cup
- Raspberries - .5 cup
- Blueberries - .5 cup

Instructions:

In a large bowl, add all of the ingredients, except for the berries, and whip them together with a hand mixer until completely smooth.

Set out four parfait glasses and divide half of the berries between all of them. Top the berries with half of the ricotta mixture, the remaining half of the berries, and lastly, the second half of the ricotta mixture.

Serve the parfaits immediately or within the next twenty-four hours.

Conclusion

Thank you for purchasing this book, and congratulations on finishing *Intermittent Fasting for Women Over* 50! I hope that through the pages of this book, you were able to gain the knowledge, understanding, and confidence you need to succeed with losing weight and gaining improved health.

While intermittent fasting may be an unorthodox lifestyle at this point, for centuries, it was a standard and everyday part of life worldwide. Not only that, but science has proven it to be both safe and effective. There is no reason to hold back from this positive lifestyle that has proven through both time and science to be such an improvement. You have everything to gain and nothing to lose by taking a step forward and making a change for the better. Whether you choose to practice intermittent fasting alone or with the ketogenic diet, you can expect to experience many benefits. While it may take a little time to adjust to the change in lifestyle, as all changes do, take heart in knowing that within a month, most people adjust and adapt.

The recipes at the end of this book will help you to stay full, satisfied, and nourished not only during your eating windows, but also your fasting windows. They are simple to follow, yet full of flavor that will keep you coming back to the dishes time and again.

You are now armed with everything you need to succeed on the road to intermittent fasting. There is no reason to hesitate. The sooner you begin, the sooner you can expect results.

Finally, if you found this book useful in any way, a review on Amazon is always appreciated!

Printed in Great Britain
by Amazon